THE WONDER WITHIN

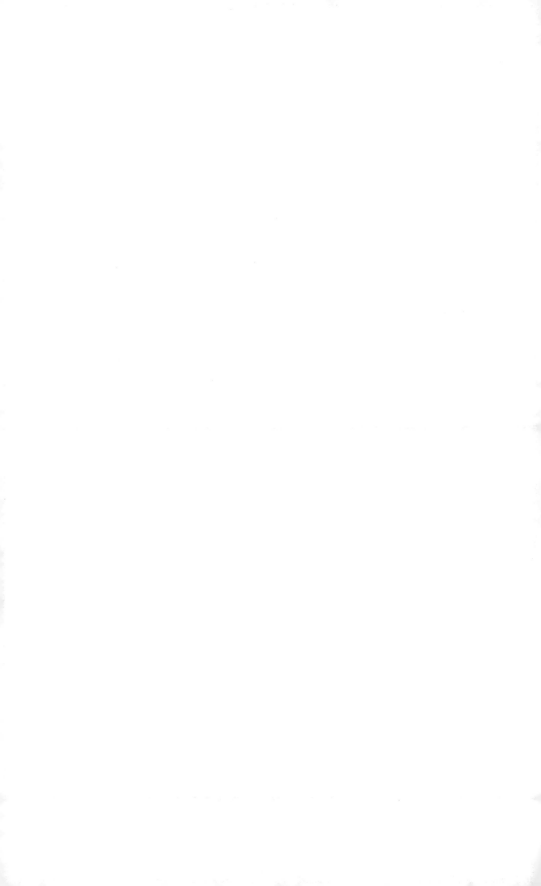

THE WONDER WITHIN

A heart-led playbook for the anxious, stressed and burnt-out

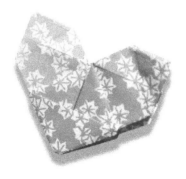

DR MICHELLE WOOLHOUSE MD

A catalogue record for this book is available from the National Library of Australia

First published in 2022 by Hambone Publishing
Melbourne, Australia

Editing by Monique Ross
Typesetting and Design by David W. Edelstein
Exercise icons by Flaticon.com

For information about this title, contact:
Dr. Michelle Woolhouse
hello@theholisticgp.com.au
www.theholisticgp.com.au

ISBN 978-1-922357-43-4 (paperback)
ISBN 978-1-922357-44-1 (eBook)

CONTENTS

ACKNOWLEDGEMENT

I respectfully acknowledge the First Nations people of Country throughout Australia, especially the traditional owners of the land where I live and wrote this book, the Boon Wurrung/Bunurong people of the Kulin Nation.

I acknowledge the cultural and spiritual connection that Aboriginal and Torres Strait Islander people have with the landscape. I am honoured to grow up here, and I am committed to learning and listening. I wish to acknowledge that this is land that has not been ceded and will always be their land.

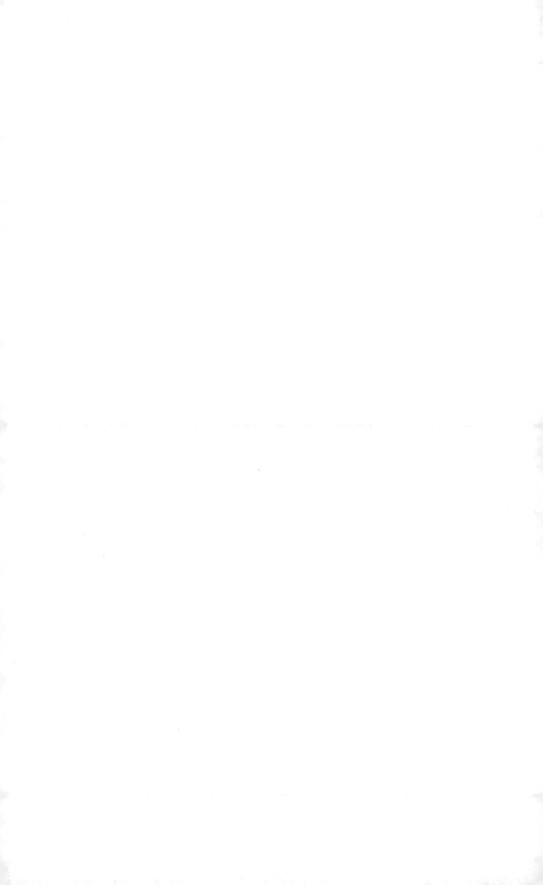

To my three greatest teachers: Will, Maggie and Lia.
From my heart to yours…
Thank you.

Wonder: (Oxford dictionary)

Noun: a feeling of amazement and admiration, caused by something beautiful, remarkable, or unfamiliar.

Verb: desire to know something; feel curious.

INTRODUCTION

"Healing is a matter of time,
but it is sometimes also a matter of opportunity."

– Hippocrates, 400BC

The human body has its own unique and innate way of healing and creating inner harmony. When you understand how this internal system works, and how to harness it, you can improve or even cure anxiety, stress and burnout, which are often offered medication as the only support. You can become an empowered player in your own health and wellbeing.

Plasticity is the scientific word for the ability to change and transform. Your experience of stress, anxiety or burnout can, if you let it, be an opportunity for change and transformation. Stress, anxiety and burnout have the power to make life so clunky, hard, uncomfortable and unsustainable that you have no choice but to find another way. They can even force a 'break down' where life has to stop, and rest, repair and recovery is the only answer.

A state of ill health or mental distress offers the chance to look within; to review your patterning, lifestyles, goals, hopes, values and ego; and to truly listen to what your body is trying to tell you. When you understand how your internal process of healing is mapped out in your body and gain greater access to your deeper self, you can use your illness and distress as a catalyst for personal growth and evolution.

This is a playbook that will give you the skills, knowledge, and inspiration to uncover your own pathway to better health and sustained calmness. It will arm you with straightforward yet powerful tools to help you work with yourself and embrace your sense of aliveness. Aliveness is a vitality that is uniquely your own. Your definition of aliveness is unique to you, and finding it will help you flourish, optimise your potential, and live with a full and open heart.

This book is also an invitation to become the artist of your health — a seriously creative process. Through modern scientific research and knowledge, alongside the wisdom of the ancients, you will learn the Art of Medicine. This occurs when a patient becomes the co-creator of their health journey. It is the magic that can spark between patient and practitioner, and it incorporates the wisdom of the person seeking health and the energetic intention of the doctor. It is a concept of the duality of medicine, and the place where science and creativity meet.

In my first week of medical school, I heard a saying: "By the time you leave, 50 per cent of what you have learnt will be wrong, we just don't know which 50 per cent." It sounds alarming at first, but medicine as an art doesn't necessarily change with each new medication or research study. Rather, the Art of Medicine grows as a doctor develops their own humanity. As Dr Francis Peabody published in the *Journal of the American Medical Association*[1], "one of the essential qualities of the clinician is an interest in humanity, for the secret of the care of the patient is in caring for the patient".

This book begins with an exploration of the holistic concepts of health: the essence of what health means, and how we are biologically built for vitality and connection. We also investigate the major players in our mindset and examine our internal and external natures to bring a sense of wholeness to our vision of health and what it means to be alive.

In Part 2, we go deeper into the body, exploring its different parts and how they interconnect to make us whole. The nervous system, the brain, the heart and the body — we break it all down into the important little details, and then build it back up again. The knowledge of how your body works is a starting point for deeper connection, and it gives you an opportunity to really own your own magnificence. I have slotted in some practical exercises to help deepen this knowledge and give you the time and space to really absorb it.

In Part 3, a guided journey begins. Through a series of exercises you will navigate the map of your own becoming, practising, building and holding onto different experiences along the way. Feel free to play around with these. Some exercises will feel natural and others may feel clunky. Some days will be easier than others. There is no right or wrong feeling. Try to approach it with curiosity and lightness. The information coming from the body can be subtle, nuanced and abstract. Practise is the only way to reveal ourselves.

It is my privilege to share my knowledge with you. I've filled these chapters with stories from my own journey and those pulled from a raft of storytellers. Some of the names have been changed and in some cases I have blended people's stories into one to make a clearer point. Throughout the book I show you ways to apply the principles of wholeness to your mind and your life. Feel free to grab a journal and work alongside the book to help you keep all your gold in one place. Where you see a little ear symbol, it means I have recorded a meditation script for you. To download the recordings or for more information and to stay connected head to www.theholisticgp.com.au.

A little note about my grammar choices; the book is written just like you are sitting in a consult, or on retreat with me. I sometimes start sentences with *And*, *But* and *Because* simply because that is how we speak and I think we need a little less formality in medicine these days.

I want to thank all the people who have supported my journey along the way: my teachers, my friends and family, my detractors, and most importantly my patients. Without you I would not have the wisdom I have today. Your generosity, your storytelling, your vulnerability and sometimes your troublemaking have helped me to grow, learn and be challenged.

Our society has normalised stress. I know from my own experience that sometimes our bodies can fight for a return to this 'normal', even though it is unhealthy and unhelpful. Change takes trust and a willingness to persist beyond the old neurology. Transformation is new-ness. It isn't just a change of jobs, or clothes or partners. If you truly want to renew and replenish your life, it takes something beyond what was there previously.

Change also takes time. Be patient with yourself as we journey together through these pages. Many of us have spent years ignoring the signs of the body and denying our feelings. It can take a while to get to know yourself and how your body communicates, and discover your sense of truth and realness.

Stress, anxiety and burnout are internal signals for change. You can become the master of your inner healing skills and use them to assist you through your medical treatment options and help you find the right health care team. Using medication during a time of anxiety, stress or burnout is a definite option, but in my opinion using them without going deeper into the causal nature of the issue is fraught with the danger of future recurrence.

Remember: you can never do yourself wrong. Even if you don't yet recognise it, you are the master of your body. You are in charge. This book, with time and practise, will allow you to know this deeply, feel it immensely and honour it truly.

We all have an innate healing mechanism. We all have deep and myste-rious parts to us. We all share the same desires for connection, belong-ing and love. This is a whole systems approach to not only health, but to aliveness. To discovering the wonder within.

part 1

DISCOVERING THE WONDER WITHIN

chapter 1

MY WHY

"It is more important to look at the person who has the disease, than the disease the person has."

– William Osler.

My anxiety started early, when I was nine years old. Impulsive thoughts no one else knew existed. Always within the silence and darkness of the night, alone and frightened. Fully trusting all that my thoughts were bringing.

I didn't come from a religious family, but I went to the local Catholic primary school. It was close to our home in the eastern suburbs of Melbourne. It introduced me to the Catechism, the dogmatic rule book of the Catholic Church. I remember being given the little green book, the size of a small notepad, and being told to keep it handy, so I could keep myself in line with God.

I was quite interested in all this God stuff, as I was a curiously spiritual little girl. I liked going to church, hearing the songs, being part of the community, the ritual and the reverence. I developed some thoughts on the matter of the Catechism, but I kept them to myself.

I was told God was all loving and all knowing. That was a little bit scary, the idea of always being watched. Then came the lesson on purgatory and hell. I wondered how this loving God could create a hell. The quickest way to get there, I was told, was by taking the Lord's name in vain. It seemed extreme.

Sure enough, a little like 'don't think about a pink elephant', that night in bed, my nine-year-old brain started silently blaspheming at God. The more my mind swore, the more scared I got. I couldn't stop. The fear grew so big I became terrified. I didn't tell anyone because I didn't want them to confirm my greatest fear: that I would be going to hell. This went on for years. My poor brain had got itself into a pickle. I found it hard to get to sleep and I was constantly worried about my descent into hell. A vicious cycle ensured. The more I tried to suppress the thoughts the more often they would come. As I became a teenager, the thoughts settled down, but the pattern — which I would only recognise many years later — had left a mark.

Exercise: Ironic Process Theory

Grab a piece of paper or your journal. I want you to do something for me as you read this next section. While you're reading, I don't want you to think about a polar bear. Don't think about it at all.

Every time you *do* think about a polar bear, mark a dash on your piece of paper.

In 1863 Fyodor Dostoevsky wrote: "Try to pose for yourself this task: not to think of a polar bear, and you will see that the cursed thing will come to mind every minute." This famous line led to a researcher, Daniel Wegner, going on to define this common thought issue as ironic process theory. Simply put, the more you try to suppress a thought, the more likely you will think it.

Wegner approached this by taking a group of people and running them through a simple task of speaking their thought stream aloud for five minutes at a time. The first time he told them not to think of a white bear, and the second time they were allowed to think of a white bear. Each time this thought came to their mind, they were to ring a bell.

The group that was told not to think of the white bear thought about it more often than those that were allowed to think about a white bear. Ironic, really.

Looking at your piece of paper, how did you go? How many times did you think about the polar bear?

In my early years of medical school my intrusive fears arose again. I was 21, and life was filled with lots of study and a few wild parties. My parents decided it was time to part ways, my sisters left home, I moved out with friends. While all this everyday life stuff was happening, my terrified brain was refusing to shut down and allow me any rest. This time my fear was about either dying or being diagnosed with one of those enduring illnesses that seemingly strikes at random: multiple sclerosis, schizophrenia, lymphoma, leukemia, bipolar disorder. The thought of an unfavourable prognosis pummelled me into a darkness which had me pinned inside my own brain, feeling utterly disempowered.

The penultimate trigger came during my placement at a now-closed psychiatric institution in suburban Melbourne. I spent every day there, interviewing all the patients from chronic psychiatric Ward 17. I was exhausted from my brain's unwelcome intrusions into my life. Seeing people who had been hospitalised for so long made my fear worse. I couldn't sleep. The slightest noise or flash of light would trigger me. I felt I was going 'crazy'.

I was then placed onto 'nights' rotation in Box Hill Hospital's Emergency Department. By this stage I was convinced that I was going crazy, but I didn't know where to turn. I was in a dark world of pain. My tears were constant. I didn't tell anyone because I couldn't put the feelings into words. I especially didn't want to tell a doctor, for fear they would confirm I really was losing it. I went on alone and without support for months. The perfect storm came as I broke up with my boyfriend. My parents were in their own emotional pain and my sisters were overseas. My whole medical future felt in doubt.

I finally went to see the doctor, revealing my darkest secrets to him. He told me I had anxiety and gave me a referral to a psychiatrist. I was shocked and felt a tinge of shame, but I timidly made an appointment. As it neared its end, I asked the psychiatrist if he thought it was safe if I went overseas. I knew I had to get away.

"This is anxiety, so it won't kill you," he said nonchalantly. A relief filled me. I gained an invitation to my life. I may have been petrified but I wasn't going to die. I was at the bottom, experiencing a dark night of the soul. I decided the only way was up.

This was the start of my foray into health and what I can now, in hindsight, call my exciting healing adventure. Over the next 30 years, I came to discover myself and my own remarkable way of recovering my mental health. I went on to not only survive but to thrive, test my boundaries, reveal my internal patterns and find my inner freedom.

I have been a GP for more than 20 years, primarily in primary care. Over time my approach has become more holistic. I have studied nutritional medicine, mind-body medicine, yoga, sound meditation, shiatsu and traditional Vietnamese acupuncture. As my approach expanded, I made room in the system for my own style. I founded an integrative family clinic, and lectured for the Australasian College of Nutritional and Environmental Medicine (ACNEM), of which I am a fellow. I also became a podcast host, and teamed up with renowned facilitator Caroline Hales to create a series of empowering wellness retreats for women.

In November 2020 I made the decision to move on from my role as owner and sell the practice. I felt a foreboding sense of burnout, perhaps accelerated by the COVID-19 pandemic and the associated issues that came along with it. Something had to change. I needed to find balance again.

The sale gave me the most precious gift of all: time. Time to rest, to lie on the grass and look up at the sky, swim, walk, surf, talk, laugh, waste away hours, read, lie in the sun and go to bed early. I didn't instantly fall into rest. It took time for my system to re-calibrate — more than I could have imagined.

I had been under the impression that as soon as I stopped to rest, I would bounce back and recover. Instant renewal, right? Nothing could be further from the truth.

Key Points:

- The more you try to suppress a thought, the more prevalent it becomes.

- Anxiety is not life-threatening.

- Recovery requires time.

chapter 2

THE BIGGEST LIE WE HAVE BEEN SOLD

"It's no measure of health to be well adjusted to a profoundly sick society."

– Krishnamurti

Our modern existence isn't set up for health. It is set up for the pursuit of money, prestige and financial success. We think that if we have enough money we will find happiness, but it doesn't work that way.

We live in the fastest paced world in human history. Things are getting busier, more rushed and more aggressive as the years go by. Stress is rife. You can hear it in the tone of voice of the barista, see it in the lack of eye contact from the ticket seller, sense it in the cursory attitude of the person at the end of the phone. We rush through life. The last time I was at yoga, the teacher said: "Enjoy these moments of stillness, before you rush out and start your busy day."

We live in a world that has no time for unwellness. We revere stress, busyness, possessions, pace, achievement, striving, persistence, success and money. The speed of modern life means we are at risk of missing its deeper aspects and therefore its meaning. We have been conditioned to fit in to this culture, to plod the regular path, to belong.

Neuroplasticity has taught us the power of change for the positive. We are told we can, through brain training exercises, relearn and adapt to problems to regain function in an area of the brain that was damaged. What we often fail to comprehend is that brain neuroplasticity is happening all the time. When we adapt to stress and get better at coping, we normalise the busyness of our lives.

In his book *The Inner Self*, renowned social psychologist Hugh Mackay writes: "One of the most curious aspects of human attitudes and behaviour is that, while we actually thrive on change and we need disruption and surprises to maintain brain plasticity and keep ourselves alert and fully alive, we constantly bemoan the impact of those changes on our lives."

We tend not to like it when people go against the grain. Society works on people doing what people did yesterday. Families work the way they always worked. Change rarely comes at a convenient time nor is it commonly welcomed by ourselves or others. But we must change, because despite all the incredible aspects of our modern life, it does not foster good health.

- There were 40.7 million prescriptions filled for mental health-related medications in Australia in 2019-20 (Australian Institute of Health and Welfare)

- Nine people per day take their own lives in Australia (Lifeline)

- 1,200,000 calls are made to Lifeline each year

- One in five teenagers has experienced an anxiety disorder (Beyond Blue)

- 25 per cent of Australians will suffer an anxiety disorder (that's about 5 million people!) (Beyond Blue)

- 46 per cent of kids have been bullied at school (Headspace)

- Anti-depressant use in people aged under 18 has increased by 60 per cent over the past five years. (Sydney University Brain and Mind Centre)

Consider also the stark rise in rates of obesity, anxiety in children, dementia and cancer, not to mention the ill health of our soils, forests, oceans and flora and fauna. This all adds up to impact not only our physical, mental and spiritual health, but the health of our society.

Australians are officially working the longest hours in any country across the world and stress levels are at an all-time high. According to the 2017-18 Australian Bureau of Statistics, an estimated 13 per cent or 2.4 million Australians aged 18 and over reported high or very high levels of psychological distress, a 12 per cent increase from 2014-15 (11.7 per cent or 2.1 million Australians). According to the American Psychological Association (APA), it is Millennials who are the worst affected. We have an epidemic of insomnia, road rage, screen-time addictions, body dysmorphia and loneliness. In 2020, the World Health Organisation (WHO) made the statement that stress is directly and indirectly responsible for more than 80 per cent of lifestyle related diseases such as heart disease, stroke, cancer and diabetes. Conditions that are made worse by chronic stress are also on the rise. Illnesses such as asthma, eczema, irritable bowel syndrome, tension headaches, chronic pain and poor attention are so common that we have normalised these maladies as a part of modern life. I have always warned patients of the obsequious acceptance of work over leisure. Many without thinking give away their holidays and pastimes in the pursuit of more work, more money and more material goods.

To feel well in a highly pressured and stressed world is no measure of true health.

Key Points:

- *You are not alone in your mental health challenges.*

- *Consider your mental health issue as a response to unrealistic pressures from our culture.*

- *We can change our brains to be both helpful and healthy or unhelpful and unhealthy.*

SEEKING REST

While stress is rife, rest is somewhat elusive. We often rest in front of the TV, or by scrolling on the internet. We rest with a glass of wine in our hand, or by going shopping. Our rest is rarely restorative. It is not purposeful, respectful nor honouring.

Katherine May is a UK-based journalist whose autism has made coping with modern stress more challenging than it is for the neurotypical general population. Her book *Wintering* is about the importance of deep and respectful rest, creating and honouring a time of fallowness in life. A time of watching, wondering, pondering and letting the process of time heal whatever needs to heal. Even though this didn't change her autism diagnosis, it made a profound difference to her sense of self, her ability to cope and her outlook on the world.

When I was a little girl, on the way home from my grandmother's house, we would pass by two convalescent homes. We would play a game of counting the number of oldies sitting in the windows, blankets over their knees, staring off into space. Convalescent hospitals were the norm up until 40 or so years ago. People would be discharged from an acute hospital to rest until their bodies were restored.

We need to do more convalescing. How can the body heal if we don't let the wisdom that wants to come forth have space and time to come?

So, I'm calling it out: busyness is the biggest lie we have been sold.

Exercise: Still Listening

Come into silence.

Now come into stillness.

Listen to your body.

Repeat steps one to three.

Note: Some people who suffer anxiety use busyness as a distraction and when they stop to rest, they feel their anxiety more. This is a very common vicious cycle, especially in women. As you work towards listening to your body, try to remind yourself that anxiety is common and treatable. But it needs to be heard and witnessed in order to transform.

chapter 3

A DISEASE MANAGEMENT SYSTEM

"The art of medicine consists of amusing the patient while nature cures the disease."

– Voltaire

The modern Western medical system is not designed as a health care system, but rather as an acute disease management system. The delivery of medicine is fragmented: we tend to treat only the system that is showing the symptoms and forego the complete picture of a person's health and wellbeing, and how this impacts the whole of their lives, their relationships and society.

Conditions such as anxiety, stress and burnout are typically managed with the quick offer of a prescription or a referral to a psychologist. When someone presents with indigestion, we treat the stomach with an antacid, but we fail to ask about their stress, their diet or their breathing. When someone presents with irregular periods, we give them the contraceptive pill, yet we don't ask about their alcohol intake, their sleep or work pressure. When someone presents with depression we give them an anti-depressant, without asking why their grief is so long lasting or what their sugar intake is or why their self-belief is low. We give antibiotics for infections, and anti-inflammatories for inflammation.

We are anti-illness, anti-exploring for the underlying cause and anti-asking if there is another way. We live in a world that is anti-feeling any discomfort. The extraordinary time pressures facing doctors, our overreliance on medications and long-held prejudices and stigmas all contribute to this.

I have met many people who believe that nothing can be done, so they do not seek help. For others it may be that because they can't see a way out of their issues, they simply assume there is no way out. Maybe their fatigue is so great, or the issues feel so immense, that the solution feels impossible. If we only have access to a 10-minute doctor's appointment, how on earth are we supposed to find the words, the meaning, and the time to explore what lies underneath our complex persona?

Whole systems of health care are not new. Ancient traditions such as Ayurveda and traditional Chinese medicine can be great teachers to Western practitioners if we open our minds and hearts to their wisdom. This book will help you understand the power of the whole for healing and why it is so important to explore a little deeper when illness and discomfort come into our lives. This deeper style of medicine can only come from those who have been intimately trained in harnessing such skills. My stress, anxiety and burnout are among my greatest teachers.

This also gives us the opportunity to work with the other systems that support the dominant system that is expressing the discomfort. For example, by working with the gut and digestive system in anxiety, we can reduce our stress and toxic load, and therefore start to feel better. We can work on the hormonal system to help alleviate stress and support sleep.

As the systems are all connected, by working on one we will affect another and vice versa. Mental health requires physical health and vice versa. By including a holistic viewpoint to every illness, we can come to view ourselves as a whole and use our illness to help us move towards wholeness.

We tend to be masters of the reductionist principles of life. We are a culture of polarisation, division and disconnection; we are obsessed with power over as opposed to power with. We learn by breaking things down, fragmenting them to understand, but we are not great at building them up again to recreate the whole. We separate mental health from physical, physical from emotional, emotional from spiritual, social from mental. We disconnect heart disease from social health, we disconnect type 2 diabetes from depression.

Holism and whole systems approaches are difficult to examine scientifically as they contain many moving parts that all affect the whole. Our current gold standard to assess health outcomes is via a reductionistic experimental approach, such as a Double Blind Randomised Placebo Controlled Trial, or DBRPCT.

In between the years 1882 and 1912 a small town in the US was formed by a large group of migrant Italians, who named it Roseto. In the 1950s, a doctor named Stewart Wolf became intrigued by Roseto and its residents, who were renowned for their longevity. No one in town had ever suffered from heart disease, despite it being on the rise almost everywhere else. Dr Wolf started to study the people of the town, measuring their physical makeup, work, diet, exercise, culture, lifestyle, cholesterol, blood pressure, weight, smoking rates and alcohol intake.

The people of Roseto did not eat excessively healthily or exercise more than the average man or woman. After years of observational studies[2], it was established that the lack of heart disease was associated with a lack of social isolation; the people of Roseto benefited from their close-knit communities, their extensive social networks and their friendships. This town that adopted the multi-generational approach from their traditional homeland provided a social inclusiveness and a sense of belonging that was not commonly found in other American towns. This became known as the 'Roseto effect' and drove home the impact of social health on our longevity and lives.

It is no surprise that recently loneliness was found to be a stronger risk factor for heart disease than smoking[3]. Well-known psychosocial researcher Robert Saplosky has found that social isolation plays a more significant role than social rank or personality in primates. "Up until 15 years ago, the most striking thing we found was that, if you're a baboon, you don't want to be low ranking, because your health is going to be lousy," he explained. "But what has become far clearer, and probably took a decade's worth of data, is the recognition that protection from stress-related disease is most powerfully grounded in social connectedness, and that's far more important than rank."

These stories ignite an understanding of the impact we have on each other's health. We are not only whole from head to toe, we are a whole ecosystem of humans, living in a togetherness that impacts our collective health. Where we live, how we live, who we commune with, how we love and how we are loved affects our blood flow, our minds, our hearts and all the bits in between. We are not isolated individuals responsible for number one, we impact each other. By understanding this we can choose whom we commune with and how we behave, and honour the effect we have on others. Taking accountability to not only look after ourselves, but humbly for the good of all.

Key Points:

- Health is based on looking after the whole system.

- No part is greater than another and the whole is greater than the sum of its parts.

- Busyness can be a risk factor for lack of connection and loneliness.

AN INNER APPEAL FOR CHANGE

Anxiety, stress and burnout express themselves in multiple ways.

Physical expressions include things like tension headaches, constipation and/or diarrhoea, lower back pain, hormonal issues such as pre-menstrual tension, menopausal hot flushes, fatigue, central weight gain, recurrent infections, cold sores, heartburn, sugar cravings and thyroid dysfunction.

Mental and emotional expressions include panic episodes, a feeling of doom, busy mind, irritability, losing your sense of humour, being easily frustrated or short tempered, or having poor focus and concentration.

These can lead to self-medication with alcohol, drugs, smoking, sweet cravings, buying things, working excessively, internet surfing, sex, and other things such as pharmaceuticals that numb the discomfort.

This is the time to get excited. Your body may be appealing to you to change, your aliveness may be wanting to be expressed. The beauty of stress, anxiety and burnout is that they offer an opportunity to revere our body's signals for health and find our way back to balance.

Often, we can miss these opportunities. We can miss the call. But we can embrace suffering and pain for simply what it is — a shared part of our collective humanity. By sharing humanity rather than hiding ourselves from it, we engage in the whole of the possibilities that the body and social set-up may be expressing. When we ignore the signs and symptoms coming from the body or from those in our lives, we tend to send the messages into repression. The body then fatigues from sending messages that fail to be received or responded to. We then risk missing the vital impetus that can inspire us to change, to head in the direction of health, be it health for ourselves or the health of the whole. Because when we heal ourselves, we inherently heal others. Just like stress is addictive and stress is collective, so too is peace and calmness. Knowing we can be whole in ourselves, we can also contribute to the wholeness of our communities. We start to commit to a new way of seeing health, life, and our place in it.

When we are dealing with such pain and suffering, it can often sideline us. Let it. This is the gold. This is the celebration. This is your body calling time out.

chapter 4

STRESS, ANXIETY AND BURNOUT

"If someone wishes for good health, one must first ask oneself if he is ready to do away with the reasons for his illness. Only then is it possible to help him."

– Hippocrates

Stress, anxiety and burnout force us to reconnect to the slower side of our lives, to the silence, the stillness. We need to hear their message so we can assess our lives, our responses, and the underlying cause of the mental unrest and dissatisfaction. Stress, anxiety and burnout are not diseases as such, they are imbalances.

Think back to the last time you felt stressed. How did you feel? Tense, angry, irritable, frustrated? Did you come down with a headache, feel spacey and foggy, or tight in the chest? Stress is a ubiquitous feeling of excessive tension or strain, felt in the body in response to a stressor. A stressor is defined as any perturbations within the system or within the environment that threaten to disrupt the organism's optimal functioning. The feeling of stress is caused by the cascade of biological processes aiming to bring the system back to balance.

It is natural to experience stress as a response to life from time to time. The body has evolved to cope with acute stressors and respond in a way that helps us to protect ourselves, stay safe and return to optimal functioning. Optimal functioning is when the body is in a state of balance. When we can ameliorate stress, our natural state of being is one of calmness and peace. In his book *The Essence of Health*, Professor Craig Hassed says: "In the relaxation response there is a move towards restoring balance, called homeostasis. This move of the body towards balance, harmony, efficiency and health is natural and will take place automatically if it is allowed. The mind too will return to happiness and contentment if it is allowed."

But the stress us modern humans experience and what we refer to in this book is chronic stress, which is not healthy for the body in any way. Chronic stress refers to a chronic overloading of the stress response system, to the point that the body naturally becomes fatigued and less able to maintain and sustain balance in all aspects of the human physiology. These physiological impacts are widespread and can be felt throughout the body, the mind and the psyche. Impacts include mental tension, emotional dysregulation, poor sleep, poor focus and poor decision-making capabilities. It also impacts the body, by dysregulating the immune system, the hormonal system and the digestive system.

Chronic stress is a modern day epidemic. We all need to take responsibility for how we respond to stress. We need to take this opportunity to look within and find our truths, and make decisions that can support ourselves and therefore the health of the whole community as well. Health starts now. Why wait?

Exercise: Life Stress Inventory

In 1967, research scientists and psychiatrists Richard Rahe and Thomas Holmes developed the Social Readjustment Rating Scale (SRRS) to identify major life stress events. They examined the medical records of more than 5,000 patients to determine whether stressful events cause illnesses. Patients ranked a list of 43 life events based on a relative score. Each event, called a Life Change Unit (LCU), had a different 'weight' for stress. The more events experienced, the higher the score; the higher the score the higher the risk of becoming ill.

There are a lot of things on the scale that we completely normalise in life these days, not recognising at all the strain these events put on us. Mostly we can all cope well with one stressor at a time, but when they accumulate the burden increases, just like tension on a string.

Take the time now to Google The *"social readjustment rating scale "*and do the online test. It lists different sources of stress, like breaking up with a partner, sickness of a child, changing jobs and moving house. As the scale was developed in 1967, there isn't a score for COVID-19 lockdowns or living through a pandemic, so we might need to take that into account too.

To work out the total value add up the scores for each event you have experienced over the year.

- A score of less than 150 means you have a 30 per cent chance of suffering from stress.

- A score of 150-299 equates to a 50 per cent chance of suffering from stress.

- A score of more than 300 means you have an 80 per cent chance of developing a stress-related illness.

What were your results?

Take a moment to reflect on your score. Perhaps you can let it inspire you even more to take the journey inward to help you discover the wonder within, which has the potential to change your response to life and help you become the best version of yourself, mentally, emotionally, physically and spiritually. Perhaps it will offer you solace, as you legitimise how much stress you have endured or are enduring.

Stress is increasing as the years progress. Research published in 2020 in the journal *American Psychologist*[4] examined the effect of stress on people aged between 45 and 64. It found a significant increase in day-to-day stress over a 17-year period.

The research looked at data from 1,499 adults collected in 1995 and compared it to 782 different adults in 2012. Both groups were interviewed daily for eight straight days. They were asked about stressful experiences they had had over the past 24 hours. Researchers found that day-to-day stress and a sense of lower overall wellbeing were considerably higher in the 2010s as compared to the 1990s. The participants in the later survey showed a 17 per cent increase in having a sense that stress would affect their future plans. They also had a 27 per cent higher belief that their financial status would be affected by stress.

We have not only normalised stress, we expect it. We have in many ways made it an unconscious habit in our daily lives. In this context stress can be seen as addictive and it can accumulate unconsciously.

Key Points:

- Stress is a vital part of our survival programming.

- Chronic stress is an overload to your innate survival code.

- Stress is more prevalent today as compared to decades prior.

- When stress levels are low the body is able to return to its innate state, which is peaceful, calm and happy.

HIDDEN STRESS

Hidden stress is stressors that come from the inside. It may be long-held unhelpful beliefs, a strong but invisible inner critic, a pesky ego or a shame filter. Hidden stress is often in people who feel strong and capable, or who don't feel understood, or feel like they are in an internal fight with themselves or the world, or have become adept at wearing the masks they were given a long time ago.

Some hints: lots of judgments, feeling disconnected, feeling like you are the only one who can be relied on, feeling like the victim, demanding things from others, sabotaging happiness or success, excessive worry, feeling responsible for everyone and everything, feeling that your needs matter less than those of others. Sound familiar?

Hidden stress manifests in the body in surprising ways and it can take some time for it to reveal itself to you. Being honest with yourself and giving yourself the opportunity to look within may help you to witness your role in perpetuating your own internal stress response.

Case Study:

Meet Helen. She has severe eczema over her face, chest, and hands. It is red and inflamed; so itchy she scratches in her sleep and wakes up with blood on the sheets. Her face feels tight and

I can tell that the eczema around her eyes makes every blink uncomfortable. She is a capable woman, in a loving relationship with three little kids. A helpful member of the community, she volunteers for the SES and works as one of the team leaders. Her husband works late and travels a lot. She does most of the housework but feels okay about it as he works hard and is tired too.

Helen has tried a dairy-free diet, a gluten-free diet, a low salicylate diet and even a mould protocol. Everything seemed to make her skin condition worse.

Helen told me she didn't feel stressed. She was the one who helped others deal with their stress. She just had to get on with it, no complaints. When I first mentioned the role of stress in the illness, she recoiled. But as she began to paint a picture of her heavy load, without judgement, blame or shame, she slowly came to allow herself some room to explore her own needs and her own emotions.

Helen is formidable, but until she could realise her limits and respect the messages that her body was trying to tell her, she couldn't regain the health of her skin. By supporting her stress and inflammation response physically, mentally, emotionally and nutritionally, her body could let go of the need for inflammation and heal itself.

Even when conditions are treated perfectly in the Western model of care, things can be missed. Most of us doctors love a cure. We love it when a person gets better and we never have to see them again. Problem gone, tick, next. But this can be an issue too — not so much for a fishhook-in-the-hand kind of problem, because accidents happen, but for conditions that warrant deeper investigation.

Case Study:

Meet Leonie. She was diagnosed with stage one melanoma after a routine skin check. It was removed, and Leonie was told to stay out of the sun, and to see a dermatologist every 12 months for review. Tick. Problem solved. But, like Hippocrates taught us, disease is either a matter of time or a matter of opportunity. If we can reframe our rather simplistic viewpoint of disease causation, and extrapolate it to include the whole person response, her early diagnosis could be more than a good luck story.

Leonie is an extremely likable, competent and successful woman who hides her stress very well. She had been stressed since childhood; she lost her father in tragic circumstances and was forced to move away from their small town and start a new life in the city. However, her mother worked hard, and Leonie thrived — until she got an immune-sensitive cancer at the age of 38. Melanoma is one of the most immune-sensitive cancers. There is growing evidence[5] to support the increasing incidence of melanoma in those with a compromised immune system and those in highly stressful occupations, alongside other known risk factors such as sunburn and genetic risk factors. Where stress is thought to be causative, shouldn't we address the impact of it in our treatment response?

Let's look at Leonie's risk factors:

- Fair skin? No.
- A history of sunburn? Only once or twice.
- Excessive ultraviolet (UV) light exposure? No.
- Living closer to the equator or at a higher elevation? No.
- Having many moles or unusual moles? No.
- A family history of melanoma? No.

Leonie did, however, have a weakened immune system, perhaps related to chronic stress. When the body is under chronic stress it releases chemicals called cytokines, which increase tumour progression.

Asking the right questions is remarked as being more important than knowing all the answers.

Leonie went on over the years to develop significant menstrual issues, a peptic ulcer, migraine headaches, and recurrent infections. She needed to look within to her patterns of striving to please and pushing at the cost of her own needs and her own health. She was outwardly successful, but her health was telling a different story.

When Leonie took the chance to go inward, despite initially feeling that this reflection was self-indulgent, she found her deeper self. Her system has found the calmness she was internally craving, yet not realising she was missing.

Our bodies don't lie. They keep the score and they tally it daily, until the game is over.

Key Points:

- Our internal dialogue, self-belief and habitual emotional patterns can be a source of hidden stress on the system.
- Stress comes from external circumstances and how we handle them, and also from the chronic pressure we put on ourselves.

ANXIETY

The felt sense of anxiety has become somewhat accepted as a part of our day-to-day lives. It's not uncommon to hear people say, "Oh, that's just my anxiety!" In decades past, we probably would have called it nerves.

Symptoms of anxiety can be varied but common experiences are feeling panicked, hot flushes, racing heartbeat, nausea or diarrhoea, feeling tight in the chest or throat, shallow breathing, agitated or feeling tense, wound up and irritable. It is common to worry a lot, make everything into a catastrophe or obsess about a thought over and over. All these feelings can result in us avoiding situations and impact our productivity and social functioning.

How does your anxiety express itself? What do you mean when you say you are anxious? Is this the same feeling as when you are stressed? What is the difference? Can you decipher your unique expression of your emotionality?

As anxiety is normalised in society, it can be easy to forget the intense and pervasive nature of the condition. Many of us experience it in short bursts, but for some people, it can define how they live and permeate their decision-making processes.

Anxiety or fear is the body's natural way of helping us to avoid danger and hopefully survive. This is how we have evolved to keep ourselves safe and protected. Fear and anxiety trigger our fight or flight response (more on this and the autonomic nervous system in Part 2). When worries and anxiety are excessive, don't go away when the threat has been removed, or become a part of your day-to-day life, this is considered an anxiety disorder.

I can't tell you how many times I have heard people refer to their anxiety disorder as something they have for life, having resigned themselves to the suffering and discomfort that goes alongside it. Acceptance is important, don't get me wrong, but acceptance that becomes resignation leaves a person open to exploitation and potentially to a life less lived.

We all have things that are outside our control, but many more within our control when we have the courage to look at our conditioning, our patterns of behaviour and the circumstances that have led us to this moment in time.

In the West we tend to see anxiety as a problem to be fixed. We do this by examining the individual and their mental and biological processes as the sole source of inquiry. By exploring how different cultures define anxiety, we can come to a different appreciation of the condition.

Indigenous and first nations people have long taken a holistic approach and view mental health to be related to the individual's emotional, spiritual, physical and mental health. They also tend to consider the individual's connection to land and to the health of their relationships. Traditional Chinese medicine[6] approaches mental health as a part of the whole body and focuses on energetic imbalances and the implications of the connections between mind, the body and the spirit.

A Japanese psychiatrist by the name of Dr Shoma Morita takes a different approach again. He says anxiety is simply excessive self-focus, and he asks patients to retrain the brain to look outward instead of inward. He talks of the concept of "the naturalness of feeling bad". In Western thinking, when we feel bad, we assume there is something wrong, something we need to fix. If we can't fix it, we tend to shame ourselves for our inadequacy. In Morita therapy, there is an acceptance that "feeling bad" is a natural part of life and by accepting this we can then choose a different way to get through it. Rather than spending time trying to work out why we are feeling or how we are feeling, Dr Morita instead encourages people to make attempts to focus on others and be helpful to themselves and to their communities. By doing this they stop trying to suppress the way they are feeling. This is not mere distraction; it is more acceptance and movement beyond.

Dr Morita says it is in the avoidance and suppression of emotions where the struggle lies. "It is a person's response and relationship to thoughts and feelings that is at the core of the problem, not the thoughts and feeling," he says. Taking the pressure off ourselves to be perfect and embracing our natural tendency to experience unpleasant feelings and irrational thoughts can help us lean into ourselves and find a new way to relate to our neurology and to the wonder within.

Anxiety is common in our culture but learning from it in a deep and holistic way isn't. Anxious thoughts will continue to come into your thought processes. The more you try to reject them, suppress them or get angry about them, the more they will come. The brain thinks, that is what it does. It is how we respond to the thoughts and how we relate to them that makes all the difference. This book with help you hold them differently. This is the way to finding more peace and more wellbeing.

Key Points:

- The more you resist your anxiety thoughts, more likely they will come.

- Acknowledging them as a part of life can help you move with them.

- In indigenous medicine, anxiety is seen as a symptom within the context of the whole; an entry point in discovering what may be disconnected and in need of support.

BURNOUT

"If you desire healing, let yourself fall ill."

– Rumi

The WHO recently committed to identifying burnout as a real and diagnosable condition, defining it as a "syndrome conceptualised as resulting from chronic workplace stress that has not been successfully managed". It is characterised by three dimensions:

- Feelings of energy depletion or exhaustion;

- Increased mental distance from one's job, or feelings of negativism or cynicism related to one's job;

- Reduced professional efficacy.

Burnout is not a condition reserved for high-flying executives or front-line health workers. It can happen to anyone. Given our current work-life culture, we are all at risk.

I developed severe burnout from 2016 to 2020, while running the medical practice. My vision was to create a group of GPs aligned to the principles of holism and integration. It was uber successful. People were coming from interstate, and we were even getting phone calls from people living overseas, wanting to get an appointment with one of our GPs. We couldn't keep up with demand. The practice quickly grew from me being the only doctor to having five GPs in the clinic.

But the pressure was immense. The expectations felt really high. Then came the crash. Over the next few months four of our doctors left. The practice had only one doctor: me. I was at breaking point, so low, so stressed, so beyond burnt out. I had red inflamed skin around both my eyes, cold sores were almost constant and I was relying on wine to settle me at night. Another dark night of the soul had arrived. I had two choices: I could fold, or I could rebuild. I chose to rebuild.

Two weeks later I received news of a grant I had been awarded. The tide turned. A whole new group of vibrant, positive doctors arrived — psychologists, dieticians, specialists and counsellors. The business was doing great, but I wasn't. Despite all my efforts — yoga, meditation, retreats, exercise, healthy food and time out — I wasn't recovering. I had gone too far. I had strived too much. I was burnt out.

During my burnout phase I realised I had forgotten what it was like to not live with stress. I was cynical, tired, wired, irritated and uptight. I had lost empathy and motivation. I was somewhat stuck between a rock and a hard place because my decision to sell the business also had stress attached. Acknowledging that I was going through a hard time, and giving myself permission to own this, helped me ask for help, get some counselling and plod along to the finish line I had put in place.

Look around you for your teachers. Sometimes they are not yet in your consciousness. It could be your illness, a doctor, a counsellor, a healer, a relative or a revered friend. If you are ready, ask your close ones for clues and support.

A NEW SENSE OF OWNERSHIP

I leaned a lot on my support network. They helped to hold me in my suffering, allowing me to connect to it, rather than finding ways to dispel it. My job was to own it, and own the choices that lead me to the situation I was in. Ownership is not self-blame, it is self-responsibility. If I didn't do this, I was at risk of being trapped in the victim mentality and potentially re-creating the issues with a different façade in the future, again and again.

I naturally take on a lot of self-responsibility, but my journey was also seeing where I wasn't responsible. I had to acknowledge that the people who betrayed me were allowed to betray me. Their job was to look after themselves and that is what they did. It was just that by doing so they let me down, and their actions created a feeling of humiliation in me. I had to learn not to take things personally. I had to own this and own my reaction to them actioning their own needs. It was becoming obvious that my job was to look after myself but surprisingly I realised I didn't know how.

In the years that followed I learned that my job is to look after myself first, and everyone else second. As much as this seems like the obvious thing to do, it was one of the hardest lessons of my life as I had no conscious knowledge that I wasn't doing it already and no conscious knowledge of what real self-compassion looked like. Looking after myself seemed like a small task, not a worthy one. Looking after myself was 'a given', yet I wasn't doing it. I thought I was looking after myself by doing yoga, exercising, sleeping well and eating healthily, but I was not giving myself psychological permission to be vulnerable, and I was putting the needs of others ahead of my own. Outwardly I was fortunate, successful, capable, intelligent, bold, courageous and wise. But I was unconsciously, ridiculously and egotistically hard on myself. My invisible personal mission was too onerous, too heavy, too big. My psyche, it seemed, had had enough of playing this game.

TRANSPARENCY

"It is only with the heart that one can see rightly; what is essential is invisible to the eye."

– Antoine de Saint–Exupery

What shocked me was how long it took me to start to feel better. I thought I would feel better as soon as the sale of the business had gone through, but it took at least three months to even feel that my neuroplasticity was renewing itself.

My brain had been so wired towards stress that I kept grasping for it even when I was resting. I was surprised how long it took to recalibrate to the new normal I was hoping for. Had I not trusted and persisted with the process of neuroplasticity, had I not trusted the need for patience, I could have been at risk of restarting a new project, diving into another stressor or creating something new too soon, before the stillness arrived, before I could tap into a new way of living. Stress felt familiar.

Accepting and seeing clearly was part of the process. Letting go of taking things personally was a large part of it. It helped me truly own me, to open up to my needs as well as those of others.

The process allowed me to watch for my tendency to blame myself. Blame is the opposite of acceptance. You can't change anything without accepting it first, respecting it second and attending to it third. Watch your tendency to blame, others and yourself. Take a deep breath when you witness this in yourself. Allow the blame to settle where it needs to, try to separate yourself from the concept of blaming and watch it, accept it and pause. Take another breath. Do this every time you find yourself blaming.

The tools and knowledge I already had inside me helped me to recover. Though it took time, being a mind-body medical practitioner I could literally watch my neurology shift, rewire and renew itself. I had to trust the process, keep up the practise and commit, even though I couldn't see my way past the darkness.

Anxiety and stress may or may not accompany burnout and vice versa, but there can be definite overlap of these three conditions. Regardless of whether you are suffering one, two or all three, you can bring new awareness to your body, your mindset and develop key skills in self-care.

Your commitment to change often lies in the small gestures of your day-to-day existence. It can be as simple as taking five minutes per day to sit in a quiet room and get to know your breath. It could be in making a commitment to starting the day with a warm water and lemon juice. In Part 3 of this book you will learn the skills to settle anxiety and stress, the stages of change and the techniques used to navigate this.

chapter 5

WELCOMING CHANGE

"Most people will do anything not to look at their souls."

– Carl Jung.

You now have an invitation to commit to the journey. An invitation to turn slightly or fully in a new direction.

Looking within, as Carl Jung says, can be unsettling. It can feel shameful. It isn't always convenient, it isn't always straightforward, and it isn't always uncomplicated. But it is an opportunity that this human life gives us.

Anxiety, stress and burnout are by their nature uncomfortable. They are a call from within that requires our attention. It is never what we want, or what we chose. We all want wellness, good health, vitality and happiness. Anxiety, stress and burnout can help us become ready.

Looking within, in my witnessing, is always fruitful, inspiring and revelatory. We come out the other side a better, wiser and more evolved human being.

But you have to be ready.

You have to be ready to face yourself. You have to want to know what lies underneath. You have to be willing to change old ways. You need to confront your shadow side.

We all have a dark side to our past. It is a natural part of this human journey. Psychiatrists call this the shadow. It is where we hide ourselves from ourselves, where we hide our macabre thoughts, our shame, our hatreds, our dislikes, our unforgivables, our anger, resentments and our injustices and our unspeakables.

It is in this dark space where some of the gold to our light will be found.

Carl Jung once said that in many cases in psychiatry, patients come bearing a wholly personal story they have never told. "To my mind, therapy only really begins after the investigation of that wholly personal story. It is the patient's secret, the rock against which he or she is shattered," he said. Our secret stories, our shadows, are the key to treatment. As Jung puts it: "In therapy the problem is always the whole person, never the symptoms alone. We must ask questions which challenge the whole."

Perhaps ask your friends if they have unspeakable secrets they haven't told any other person. Shame they have never shared. They don't have to share them, but just by asking, you will know that you are not alone.

IT TAKES COURAGE

"It takes courage to live through suffering,
and it takes honesty to observe it."

– C.S. Lewis

Courage is the antidote to fear. The word comes from the French word 'coeur' which means heart. In my experience and in the science, looking towards the heart, seeking out its wisdom, brings the most depth to your healing journey. It is where you find your truth, your sincerity, your self-compassion and your authenticity. It is the lifeblood of your sense of aliveness.

You need to have courage to sit with your discomfort, your fear, your pain. This is very hard to do alone, but you will learn and embrace some skills to do this in Part 3 of this book.

You must have the courage to be open to the wisdom of the body. In my experience, the internal mysteries of the body and how we individually hold our painful stuff is unique. What isn't unique is that we all have stuff to deal with. We all have unmet needs. These unmet needs may come from trying to fit into a family that had different needs, or from other formative relationships. Traumatic events such the death of a close family member, mental illness in the family, or the pain of your parents' divorce can cause a significant impact. Events we experience as children and adolescents tend to shape the person we become in our adult life. Experiences like changing schools, bullying, suffering sexual or emotional abuse, or feeling neglected by caregivers who were never home. These types of experiences and feelings can leave you with emotional needs that, even after years, have not been met. Sometimes it is a case of being a sensitive person born into a more robust family or vice versa.

There are two parts to growth: belonging and authenticity. Our need to belong is a biological imperative. If we don't belong, we don't survive. We are wired for connection and love. But we aren't always 'loveable' and there is no such thing as a mother or father or caregiver who doesn't have bad days, or who at times needed to tend to the needs of people other than their child. Most of us will arrive in adulthood with unmet needs, some more than others. This is not victim blaming or shaming of parents. It is simply a reflection on the human journey.

The other aspect of the human journey that is inherent in all of us, and shines so brightly throughout those teenage years, is individuation and authentic expression of who we truly are. However, being authentically ourselves is not necessarily convenient all the time, when there are societal conditions and unwritten rules in the family to adhere to so that control is not lost. Many families run to the beat of a cultural norm, and when it comes time for the teenagers to individuate and find their own independence this can cause disruption. Depending upon the family, there may or may not be room for this disruption. If there isn't room within the family construct this can mean the individuation is not respected and is at risk of being quashed, rejected or shamed.

Many people find their authenticity is shunned. It feels inconvenient. This can lead to burying those parts of yourself that are required for an optimised expression of your own aliveness. This reproach can lead to conflict between our two biological-social imperatives. To belong or to be authentic? Ideally, we should never have to make a choice, but many don't have this option.

BE PATIENT

"Patience is the way to joy."

– Rumi

This is a story told by a writer called Lettie Cowman, who travelled to Africa more than 100 years ago.

There was a group of European missionaries serving in Africa a century or so ago. They needed to hire a group of local villagers as porters to help carry supplies to a distant station. The porters went at a slower pace than the missionaries desired, so after the first two days, they pushed them to go faster. On day three of the trek, the group went twice as far as day two. Around the campfire that evening, the missionaries congratulated themselves for their leadership abilities. But on day four, the workers would not budge.

"What's wrong?" asked one missionary.

"We cannot go any further today," replied the villagers' spokesman.

"Why not? Everyone appears well."

"Yes," said the African, "but we went so quickly yesterday that we must wait here for our souls to catch up with us".

In the past, patience was seen as a virtue; a way of understanding that life actually has a sense of timing to it; that there is an innate intelligence; that it can't be rushed; that waiting for the timing to be right is a sign of wisdom. Our modern world is bereft of patience. We rush through, admiring speed as the only way forward. By coming into the subtle intelligence of patience we can support and oppose this inane, disease-manifesting aspect of modernity.

Our modern medicine is also a victim of this faster pace. We want a quick fix as patients, so we turn to medications. Doctors get paid more for seeing more patients, so appointment times have shrunk. Our whole culture is the antithesis to the way of nature. Nature is cyclical. Its features are growth, contribution, rejuvenation, death, wintering, springing forth, losing and renewing. Our Western world has done away with rest.

Anxiety, stress and burnout are prime examples of what happens when we are out of balance, when work and the mind are too busy, when our load is too much to bear. To acknowledge this is brave, to acknowledge we have gone too fast over our lives is wisdom.

Key Points:

- We all have a shadow side, internal shame, things we find unbearable or unforgivable.

- We all arrive at adulthood with unmet needs.

- Patience, courage and sincere effort are required for the journey within.

- We all need to find the right balance between individuality and belonging.

A NON-LINEAR JOURNEY

"Nothing ever goes away until it has taught us what we need to know."

– Pema Chodron

Readiness to look within does come in stages, and self-knowledge is done at your own pace. You can stop any time, take a pause —you are in total control. As you go through the exercises in this book, you may feel a sense of calm, you may feel more stressed, you may feel nothing at all. Each time you do an exercise, hold your patience, hold your resistance, and hold your integrity.

Doing things for the first time can feel boring, pleasant, scary or completely weird. These are all normal experiences. But if you feel like you want to develop a deeper relationship with yourself, find your own sense of mastery and become more in charge of who you are, then courage, repetition, patience, practise and curiosity are the key attributes to bring along for the ride.

Watching your self-judgement, your self-criticism and your resistances brings information that can be critical to moving forward in your well-being journey. Know you are not alone in these issues, almost everyone I have met and taught share them with you. You may have issues deep within you, patterns that you have carried, or a sense that your true self is not worth the light of day.

The journey to whole, to truth, to the heart, is never a straight line. It isn't without confusion. But without this journey you are settling for less: being less than you can be, being less alive, and being less than whole.

Exercise: Finding Your Why

Take a minute, just to sit quietly and reflect. Ask yourself: 'What do I want and why? What do I want to improve on? What is my ultimate goal? Why is this something I desire or long for?

It could be that you want to be happier, to reduce your stress load, find your peace, feel free. See what comes, when you simply ask yourself what you want.

If nothing comes immediately or clearly, see if you can be patient with yourself, allowing some space in your mind's eye for reflection. You may find that by simply asking the question is enough to set off a line of inquiry that will ultimately be supportive of a deeper part of yourself that is rarely, if ever, expressed.

chapter 6

THE IMPORTANCE OF HOLISM

"Humankind has not woven the web of life. We are but one thread within it. Whatever we do to the web, we do to ourselves. All things are bound together. All things connect."

– Chief Seattle 1854

In medical school I was proficient in four subjects: neurology, psychology, immunology and endocrinology (the hormonal system). My fascination in these areas far exceeded the other systems of the body. So, you can imagine how excited I was when I signed up for the post-graduate diploma in psycho-neuro-immunology. Since then, the combination of triads has grown, to psycho-neuro-endocrinology, psycho-neuro-cardiology and even psycho-neuro-spirituality.

I'm not making these up. The field of science is carving its way towards what the ancient, traditional and indigenous cultures have lived by all along. We may like to think one part of the body has power over the other, but it is power within not power over that is the guiding principle of nature and therefore of humanity.

These sciences of the whole are catching up, but wholeness will never be validated by the gold standard randomised controlled trials that most doctors will need to have to bring them into modern medicine. Even though many of us, including doctors, intuitively know the holistic nature of our beings, it is still a challenge to confront this within our conservative culture and especially within our modern medical system.

Contemplation through whatever means can allow us to incorporate our own uniqueness into our universal neurology and collective psychology. This eludes the realms of scientific application. Our lives are not a uniform science experiment, thankfully. It is our inner and outer culture, beliefs, dispositions, experiences, stories, fears, patterns, interpretations and shames which are unique to us. This is where medicine is an art, informed by science. It is not a pure science and it never will be.

In his book *The Inner Self*, Hugh Mackay explores the issues that can occur when either science and religion narrow by putting too much value on each at the expense of other branches of learning and culture. When this occurs, it is called fundamentalism or scientism. Dr Mackay says "at its extreme, scientism claims that science is the only valid source of knowledge — the same claim religious extremists make for religion". French philosopher Bruno Latour, in his book *On the Modern Cult of the Factish Gods,* makes the claim that scientists are at risk of making leaps of faith, just like religious zealots do.

They do this through their own internal bias, beliefs, culture and seeing facts as ultimately stable, when they are, like many things, subject to change and re-interpretation as new understandings come to light. Science is a very important part of medicine, but it is not the only influencing factor in healing, health and our expression of our own aliveness. Science, like religion, is open to being revised or reinterpreted when new research or understanding is uncovered at a later time.

Key Points:

- Science is an important part of medicine, but it will never be the only source of knowledge in patient care.
- Personal meaning, interpretation, connection and wholeness are critical aspects of the human journey and of health.

THE PLACEBO EFFECT

"A doctor, like anyone else who has to deal with human beings, each of them unique, cannot be a scientist: he is either, like the surgeon, a craftsman, or, like the physician and the psychologist, an artist."

– WH Auden

We get some inklings of our uniqueness when we come to explore the placebo effect, which all scientific applications acknowledge and utilise within the modality of research guidelines.

Placebo is Latin for 'I will please'. It applies to any medical treatment that has no active properties. Placebos are often used in clinical trials for new treatments. It doesn't have to be a pill. It can be any treatment, such as injecting water, doing dummy acupuncture or even sham surgery.

In 1959, a surgeon named Leonard Cobb was perplexed as to why a procedure called "internal mammary artery ligation" actually worked. The surgeons opened the chest and then closed one of the main arteries close to the heart to force other arteries to dilate. The patients reportedly said they felt less chest pain, more energy and could go on with their lives. But despite feeling better, the procedure didn't reduce their risk of having a heart attack at a later date.

Dr Cobb intuitively felt there was something inherently wrong with the procedure. The next 40 patients who came to him complaining of chest pain and breathing difficulties were divided into two groups. On one group, he did the internal mammary artery ligation procedure. In the other group he simply opened the patient up, did nothing and closed them back up again.

The results were extraordinary — 73 per cent of the people who received the ligation procedure recorded feeling better. But in the group that received the "sham surgery" a whooping 80 per cent felt better.

These results sent shockwaves through the medical world. Not only did it lay to rest the internal mammary artery ligation procedure, which was ineffective in the long-term, but it opened the minds of the profession to the potential of the power we have inside our own minds.

The placebo effect is the positive outcome on a person's health that occurs after taking a placebo. It is influenced by a person's belief that the treatment will bear benefit and via their expectations of feeling better, rather than the influence of the placebo itself.

The placebo effect is often touted to be around 40 per cent, but can be higher when the doctor-patient relationship is strong, when the doctor has faith in the treatment and when the patient has had a family member or friends have good results from seeing the doctor in the past. It also seems that the more invasive and seemingly dangerous surgeries in the minds of the recipients, the better the effect. Even getting a needle or receiving a placebo intra-venously has a greater effect than giving it orally.

It is still somewhat of a mystery as to exactly how the placebo effect works. Some of the theories include:

- Change in motivation: the person who is seeking treatment is motivated to make a change in their behaviour. Therefore, the placebo may increase a person's conviction to take better care of themselves, such as improving their diet, starting a regular exercise program or increasing their rest. This may result in a better outcome.

- Altered perception: the person's understanding of their symptoms may change as they expect or hope to feel better.

- Reduction in anxiety: taking the placebo, combined with expecting to feel better, may alleviate the stress associated with being unwell, such that the stress chemicals like adrenaline settle, and add to the reduction in symptoms.

- Alteration in brain chemicals: the placebo may trigger the release of the body's own natural pain relieving chemicals, such as endorphins.

- Alteration in brain state: research shows that the brain responds to an imagined scene in a very similar way as it responds to an actual real-life scene. It is proposed that the placebo may help the brain to recall a time before the symptoms began, and this then brings a change to the body. This theory is called 'remembered wellness'.

Other factors involved in an increased placebo effect include:

- The features of the placebo: if the pill looks authentic, the person taking it is more likely to trust that it contains medicine. Research shows that larger pill sizes suggest a stronger dose than smaller pills and taking two pills seems to be more effective than swallowing just one. Injections have a more potent placebo effect than pills.

- The person's attitude: if the person expects the therapy to work, the chances of a placebo effect are greater, but placebos can still work even if the person is doubting the effectivity. The power of suggestion is at play in this situation.

- The doctor-patient relationship: if the person trusts their health care practitioner, they are more likely to believe that the placebo will work. If the doctor believes the placebo will work, this also has a greater influence on the outcome in a positive way.

If a combination of the above is at play, say the patient trusts the doctor, the doctor trusts the treatment, and the doctor has successfully treated other people or family members that the patients know, the placebo effect can be up to 80 per cent of the positive benefits that a patient achieves.

THE NOCEBO EFFECT

The nocebo effect is an often-forgotten phenomenon in the world of medicine. The term nocebo comes from the Latin 'to harm'. It is the reverse of the placebo effect and applies in situations where a negative outcome happens due to a belief that the treatment will cause harm.

Nocebo suggests that patients are more likely to experience an adverse outcome if they anticipate or are anxious about an adverse effect. Adverse effects can be physical experiences and are often clinically diagnosable, such as nausea and vomiting in chemotherapeutic trails. Many experts think the nocebo effect has a greater effect on clinical outcomes than the placebo effect, as negative perceptions are moulded faster than positive ones.[7]

The nocebo effect can be influenced by 'media storms' and widespread broadcasting of concerns about an adverse reaction to a medicine, which has been seen to lead to an increase in the number of negative outcome reports. For example, in 2013 British media highlighted the adverse effects, including muscle pains, of a drug that is used to lower cholesterol, collectively called 'statins' following an article that was published in the *British Medical Journal*. An estimated 200,000 patients stopped taking statins within six months of the article, many due to adverse reactions. The physical symptoms have in part been attributed to the nocebo affect.

Things such as cheaper medicines, plain packaging, generic branding, close family members opinions and social media have also been associated with an increase in the nocebo effect.

We have more power on how life impacts us than we realise. By understanding the validity of both placebo and nocebo we can acknowledge the power of belief and the power of trust. What and who you trust and believe is up to you. This is your unique quality. We often go through our lives not questioning ourselves, our conditioning or our patterns and therefore are at risk of leading lives that are un-pondered, un-explored and vulnerable to the whims of powerful influences that may not have our best needs at heart.

The placebo and nocebo effect help us wake up to how we work as a system. By trusting ourselves we become players in our health. It helps us to realise how much influence we have over ourselves and can open us up to new possibilities in the landscape of our lives.

Key Points:

- Both the placebo and nocebo effects play an important role in the effectiveness of any health care intervention.

- Becoming a proactive part of your own health journey can allow you more influence over the outcomes.

WAKING UP

"The most beautiful thing we can experience is the mysterious."

– Albert Einstein

In 1995, Professor David Sackett coined the term evidence-based medicine (EBM), which was to form the basis of all medical decisions. It includes the clinician's expertise, the patient's culture and beliefs, and the best scientific knowledge available.

This has been one of the most subtle and important movements in modern medicine. It has eluded the eyes of the public and polarised medicine from an art form to a reductionistic linear approach. Measurability and metrics are very important in health care, but medicine has become focused on the science that can be measured, at the expense of other aspects that are innately human.

Having finished medical school, a shell of my former self, I was on the edge of a nervous breakdown. Fragile, fearful and anxious. One of my first placements was in the infectious diseases ward at the Alfred Hospital in Melbourne's inner east. I was fascinated by the role of bacteria and viruses and how they manifest in sometimes the most bizarre ways. HIV and the AIDS epidemic was still in full swing, and watching this virus attack the immune system was a fascination to me. But the reality of this illness was a tragedy of such a scale it was overwhelming. Trying to put a needle in the arm of a severely emancipated man, on the edge of death, was terrifying. Watching young men die alone in their rooms was horrifying. As a 23-year-old, I didn't have the capacity nor the support to cope.

In desperation, I booked into the Holistic Health Conference in Lorne in 1999, to find a solution to this overwhelming feeling of dread, fear and lack of meaning. The weekend was a turning point for me.

I went to a lecture by Professor Ian Brighthope, an incredible orator, who waxed lyrical about how he had witnessed the resolution of a young man's psychotic thinking within three days of starting a water fast. I was blown away. Never in my eight years of medical training had I heard any mention of the relationship between food and mental illness. He spoke then of the common stressors within our diets that can lead to an increase in anxiety and depression — sugar, caffeine, alcohol, food chemicals, dairy and wheat. Not only that, when illness is rife, such as at times of infection, anxiety and inflammation, the body utilises more nutrients than when it is well. Replacing these nutrients can help speed up the recovery and bring back balance into the body.

To have this intervention emphasised and explained revolutionised my understanding of illness and utilising the body's innate healing to exacerbate recovery. I came home feeling the most positive I had for a long time. I set about to stop caffeine, sugar, food chemicals and alcohol all at once. I discovered, within a week, the power of changing the inner 'milieu' of my body to settle the overwhelming mess of my mind.

The results for me were outstanding. I slept better, I had more energy, I felt positive and empowered. Those intrusive recurring negative thoughts decreased and my anxiety somewhat settled. Little did I know what I was doing in a holistic sense, but it started the journey to understanding these interconnections and how by embracing the whole we can truly transform our own health, both physically and mentally.

By focusing on my physical health, I found a tremendous transformation in my mental health, and along the way discovered a huge reservoir of gold by embracing the whole. But the converse is also true for those who suffer with physical ailments. If we fail to look towards the mind and brain and the whole nervous system to aid in our recovery, we potentially miss a huge treasure trove of wisdom and healing.

Exercise: The Calmest Version of You

Set a timer for 15 minutes. Put on a piece of music that you love. Get comfortable, warm and cosy. Simply sit back and take a breath. Try to visualise yourself feeling the calmest you have ever felt.

You might visualise yourself somewhere in nature, or at your favourite spot. Find yourself a space to be peaceful and safe. If you're not great at visualising, simply imagine it instead. And if you can't get there either, simply focus on your desire for peace, relaxation and calmness.

Consider yourself being whole. Acknowledging the physical body, the mental and emotional aspects of your brain and your inner spirit. Let the music help you resonate with the wholeness of being you.

OUR INNER MYSTERIES

"Everything is energy and that's all there is to it. Match the frequency of the reality you want and you cannot help but get that reality. It can be no other way. This is not philosophy. This is physics."

– Albert Einstein

Stress, anxiety and burnout often make you feel as if you are a bit player in your life, like you lack control, like you lack choice. The wonder within tells a different story.

Your illnesses can help you wake up to the wonder and mystery of this lived life. You are a part of this great wonderland called life. You are not above it, nor do you control it, but you are inherently connected to it, and the lives of others.

We have all experienced coincidences in life, those moments that become like folklore in our lives. One of my incredible synchronicities occurred on the eve of the birth of my second baby. I was 10 days out from the due date and there had been no signs of anything to speak of. My husband was going to collect some birth equipment we had hired from our midwife and as he was driving to her house, my daughter Maggie, two-and-a-half years old, stated very clearly: "Baby coming tonight."

"Tonight?" my husband asked.

"Baby coming tonight," Maggie repeated.

Sure, enough at 11.30 pm, it began. Baby Lia arrived the next morning as the sun rose, 10 days before she was due.

Coincidences are in everyone's lives. Mathematicians and other statisticians put them down to chance occurrences and that may very well be the case. The term synchronicity was coined by Carl Jung in the 1950s to explore the interconnections of coincidences in people's lives and how to use them to affect people's consciousness. In realms beyond science, consciousness is seen as an energy that pervades all things, from humans to animals, insects, bacteria, trees and rocks. It is what connects us all and is referred to as 'one-ness' in most traditional religions.

Trees communicate using the same hormones and amino acids that we use in our human neurology. Sharks communicate using electrical sensors in their skins; forests are one ecosystem, using vast tracks of fungi to support interconnections and for survival.

Coincidences helps us to define meaning, and they are thought to be more common in the lives of those who consider themselves spiritual. It is clear that we don't know everything and that rationality, statistics and science provide an incomplete view of the universe and our reality.

What we do know is that energy is real, it's just that science can't hang its hat on it, as it seems to go beyond our black-and-white rational thinking. Science can't seem to process what all that means in our lives. If there is an energetic connection between us and the world, would we all be choosing to live the lives we are living? Exploring energy and synchronicity allows us to open to possibilities of new perspectives in life. This is your life and you are the major player in the wonder that you create and behold. You can determine whatever meaning you want from life. You can see serendipity in a rational light or you can play around and search for more meaning if you want to.

It may seem daunting, but it is an important part to understanding the very nature of healing. By engaging in this, you will better understand the power you have within your own life to make the changes and move toward being fuller, more whole and more alive.

Exercise: Vitally You

Imagine, visualise or desire yourself laughing, feeling free, having vitality again, taking a risk, feeling adventurous, see yourself connecting with those you love, having the courage to lean in and ask for what you need.

Imagine yourself feeling abundant joy. Where are you? What are you doing? Where do you feel it inside you? What does it feel like in your body?

Key Points:

- Energy, how we make it, use it, exchange and respect it, is a critical part of owning our own health journeys.

- Opening up to energy can help us to find new meaning in our reductionistic ways of thinking.

chapter 7

QUANTUM PHYSICS

"There is no nothingness — with these little atoms that run around too little for us to see. But, put together, they make something. And that to me is a miracle."

– Mary Oliver

Put simply, quantum physics describes how everything works. It describes the nature of the particles that make up matter and the forces with which they interact.

Quantum physics underlies how atoms behave, and therefore why chemistry and biology work as they do. We all work intimately with quantum physics every day, without realising it. For example, it explains how electrons move through a computer chip, how photons of light convert to electrical currents in a solar panel or amplify themselves in a laser. It is also how synchronous events between two human beings work.

Niels Bohr, one of the fathers of quantum physics, said: "Everything we call real is made of things that cannot be regarded as real. If quantum mechanics hasn't profoundly shocked you, you haven't understood it."

Most people who aren't into science are timid to enter the realm of quantum science or energy medicine. I want to try to engage you in this, as I believe it is imperative that you enter this wonderous side to science. It can be the impetus to open your mind to your potential.

There are three main concepts I would like to explore with you.

1: Time and space, energy and matter, phenomena and their observers, everything is interconnected, according to modern physics.

One of the most revolutionary concepts that Albert Einstein is famous for is his theory of relativity, which found that time and space are interdependent. Because light takes time to reach our eyes, the further away an event is from us, the later we see it. Time became the fourth dimension of our formerly three-dimensional space. It is not possible to speak of space without speaking of time too, and vice versa. They exist only in connection with each other and simply cannot be separated.

Einstein also discovered that matter and energy are simply two different aspects of the same reality. This is the precise meaning of his legendary formula $E = mc2$. It means any amount of energy can be denoted as a certain mass at a certain speed and vice versa. Take the example of light. Isaac Newton discovered that light was made of small photon particles and another person called Christiaan Huygens discovered that light was an energy source.

Subatomic physics has now revealed that if you observe something at a quantum level, just by observing it, you connect with it, in a way becoming a part of the scene. In quantum mechanics, there's no such thing as an outer observer. As soon as you observe, you become.

Take a moment to sit with this. This is fundamental to understanding how our perception of life shapes our life. What we pay attention to grows. If we pay attention to hate, anger and separation, we limit our observation of love, integrity and peace. A fundamental principle of indigenous wisdom becomes grounded in science via the pathway of quantum physics.

2: Movement and change are constant behaviours of the universe.

In 1929, astronomer Edwin Hubble discovered that the universe was born around 10 billion years ago, from an explosion called the Big Bang. Since then, it has kept slowly expanding and some scientists think its movement is never going to stop. Movement is a fundamental rule for all entities big and small, from planets, to humans, to subatomic particles.

The inner features of an atom are protons, neutrons and electrons. All these only exist in movable structures. Particles constantly emerge and subside, energy patterns flow, ceaselessly changing from one form to another.

When the movement is very slight and stable, atomic particles are seen to us. This is the matter we see in our everyday lives. Even though things like a table and chairs seem still, the atoms in them are in constant motion. They're never still. They keep oscillating rhythmically.

To frame it another way, Einstein's renowned equation shows us that matter turns into energy and energy into matter. It is simply a continuous cycle of movement.

Of itself, energy is also a form of movement in the shape of waves and particle vibrations. Evidently and invisibly, our universe never stops dancing.

Exercise: Dancing Stardust

Take a moment to tune into your own body right now. Your cells dance alongside the beat of your heart all day long. You are a moving, expression of the universe. You and everyone else you know. We are all dancing pieces of stardust! Incredible, isn't it?

Let this sink in. Please don't pass over this quickly because the insights and the intimacy that can come from this are extraordinary. I don't want you to miss it.

3: Eastern wisdom has recognised reality as oneness and dynamic energy for thousands of years.

Some indigenous cultures, like the First Nations people of Australia, have traditions and philosophies that have lasted for at least 60,000 years. Other well-known traditions, such as Hinduism, Buddhism and Taoism, date back thousands of years to India and China.

One of the key ideas of Hinduism is Brahman, which denotes the inner essence of all things. It fundamentally views the world as an ever-changing reality, where things and their interconnections continuously evolve. It is said that the highest spiritual state one can attain in Hinduism is liberation. It occurs when you feel the oneness and the constant movement. However, liberation is not something you can attain by using rationality. You achieve it by developing your perception, through, for example, the practise of yoga and meditation.

Buddhists also believe in the unity of everything and suppose that our persistent belief in seeing ourselves as separate from the whole is the cause of our suffering, discomfort and lack of ease in this lived experience of life. They also acknowledge the ever-changing nature of reality and call this impermanence. Their underlying way of life, called Dharmakaya, is underpinned by acknowledging the premise of oneness and impermanence as part of the fundamental principles of life.

Incredibly, thousands of years ago the Taoist master Lao Tzu taught his students that an energy pervades and unites everything. He called it the Tao, or "the way". This concurs with the Hinduist Brahman and the Buddhist Dharmakaya. The Tao also acknowledged the underlying dynamic forces. "Returning is the motion of the Tao" and "going far means returning," said Lao Tzu in the 7th century BC.

Quantum physics is the possible linkage of the ancient wisdom with modern scientific methods. One of last century's greatest physicists, Werner Heisenberg, said: "In the history of human thinking the most fruitful developments frequently take place at those points where two different lines of thought meet." Albert Szent-Gyorgyi, a Nobel prize winner and biochemist, stated: "In every medical tradition before modern Western medicine, healing was accomplished by moving energy."

Listening to the words of lauded physicists, spiritual leaders and renowned geniuses is arguably a humble way to redefine what healing can mean for us. Our modern science is revealing that we are both energy and matter, we are discovered in our state of witnessing, we have endless potential for change, and we are intimately connected to the oneness of life and the impermanent nature of the universe. I know, right? Quantum physics is a total wow!

Not only can it be mind-altering, but it can open up our potential to connect within ourselves, and also to the inner potential of others and the incredible depth of indigenous wisdom. It is a gateway to helping us to dismantle our ignorance, our arrogance and our small-minded approach to illness. Once opened the gateway offers us endless opportunity to embrace a wider view of the world and our place within it.

Exercise: The Wonder Meditation

Ideally this meditation is done outside. If it is available to you try to find a beach, a park or a mountain-top. It can be done at dawn, dusk or under the night sky.

Take a moment to focus on your breath. Bring in the wonder of the possibility of being at one with this crazy mind-blowing experience we all call life. Breathe it in. Breathe in the wonder. Stay with it. You might feel a little strange doing this at first, but give it a go. Give yourself the experience of feeling the wonderful nature of nature itself.

Look around you with wider eyes. The chair you are sitting on is a moving vibration of life; the trees are all in on this too. The sun, the moon, the grass. They have the same energy flowing through them as you do.

In your mind's eye, bring in some of the people who you love. Imagine this energy and vibration running through them. Does it let you think a little more broadly? Explore your thinking, widen it, broaden it, make it bigger. Expand your world, expand your mind. You are a wild mixture of biology, chemistry, physics, energy, vibrations and synergy.

You've got this. You own it, this is yours, this is ours. This is our connection to ourselves, each other and life itself. This is the opportunity to wow ourselves, to search for our potential in small and bigger ways.

Breathe in the wonder, let your heart and breath expand inside you. Let your mind grow in new ways. Breathe. Breathe. Feel it. Feel the wonder inside you.

Key Points:

- Understanding quantum physics gives you the opportunity to understand that healing is a constant opportunity, through movement, energy exchange and connection.

- Everything is interconnected.

- Movement and change are a constant.

- The concept of oneness is a part of every indigenous culture.

chapter 8

THE WHOLE ECOLOGY OF LIFE

"You don't need another person, place or thing to make you whole."

– Maya Angelou

Quantum physics is not the only way to perceive the interconnection of life that we all share. For a mixture of reasons, the Western world has chosen division, polarisation and reductionism to be the framework of our society. Despite many people and systems adhering to the ideas of holism, our fragmented way of thinking has left a mark, and has resulted -perhaps unintentionally- in an overriding sense of separateness and competition.

If we look at the science of environmental ecology which underpins our biology as a species, we can see how important interconnection is. The Cambridge Dictionary defines ecology as the relationship of living things, including human beings, to their environment and to each other. We breathe in oxygen that the trees make and breathe out carbon dioxide in return for them to take their next breath. Just like the bees help the plants spread their pollen far and wide and the pollen feeds the bees and helps them make honey. Reciprocity, mutuality and interbeing is at the heart of the natural world.

Actions, behaviours, habitats, food choices, farming, forests, and more are all interrelated in the web of life. How we interrelate inside ourselves is replicated in how we interrelate outside ourselves. We do not only interrelate in the present. What we have done in the past relates to the present and then into the future — not just for this generation, but for future generations as well. We are biologically, energetically, ecologically, and physiologically driven by and for connection.

We are more than human; in fact, some people comment that we are more bacteria than we are human. Over the past decade there has been an explosion of research into the importance of the health of the ecosystem inside our guts, on our skins, in the vagina and in breast milk. Diversity, adaptability and balance are the vital underlying principles in health of these ecosystems.

As I was discovering this landscape of incredible wonder, I met a permaculture ecologist called Martin Sacker. Martin was a guest on my podcast The Good Doctors back in 2015, and he talked about the importance of the bacteria in the soil for the growth and nutrient density of the fruits and flowers of the plants. He explained how soil bacteria communicate to the fruit and/or flower of the plants via their messaging system and flow of the energetics within the stems.

Fascinated by this, the following week we interviewed another professor, this time of nutritional medicine. Luis Vittetta talked about the way the gut bacteria communicate to all the various organs in our bodies, how the gut bugs talk to the pancreas in order to influence the amount of digestive enzymes required, or to the liver or to the spleen.

These fascinating advanced communication synergies are all working silently inside us. Perhaps acknowledging this wonderland could give us more inspiration and motivation to consider ourselves intricately in sync with the lifeforce that is constantly at play in the inside and outside world. In Part 2 we will drill down further into the systems that play their part in the welfare of the whole.

OUR CHEMISTRY

Another fascinating way to look at our interconnections is to explore our chemistry. The invisible world of chemistry is where we exchange and interchange chemicals from within our bodies to outside our bodies. I'm not talking only about kissing here, but instead about the very makeup of our cells.

We are energetic creatures but when we look at our chemistry we are made up of elements from the universe; made up of things like hydrogen, carbon, nitrogen, magnesium, and oxygen. In fact, the atoms in your body were born inside a star.

To blow your mind even further, as the universe was formed, it was made up of hydrogen. It wasn't until some stars blew up and transformed hydrogen into other elements such as oxygen and iron that the planets were formed. Millions of years later life was formed, and then humanity. Remember the exercise we did on page 66? You are quite simply made up of stardust, and the atoms currently inside you will be made into stars again.

Exercise: Universal Connections

The next time you can, under the cloak of darkness, take some time to look upwards to the stars. Do yourself a favour and wonder at the moon. Imagine your body being made of the same elements of the twinkling stars. How does it feel to sense the connection with this vast universe, rather than just looking up fleetingly? Ponder longer, so that the pondering allows you to take ownership of your own wondering. Stay as long as the night sky allows you. Let the wonder permeate inside your body. Breathe it in and reflect how you feel. This is a representation of how incredible you are, and how incredible the world is.

As we breathe in oxygen from the air, this combines with glucose from our diet. Glucose plus oxygen produces carbon dioxide, water and energy in our cells. Oxygen that has been inside my body may be the same atom of oxygen that is currently inside your body. You might have the same atom of oxygen that was inside Einstein's living body, or that of a Tyrannosaurus Rex. We are linked by our chemistry, which is constantly changing and moving in and out of our bodies, sharing these elements with those both alive and dead.

Another amazing aspect of our health and life force is that it doesn't energetically stay within the confines of the skin. Our skin is a permeable membrane, meaning we can absorb things through our skin and we can release chemicals via the skin too. More than sweat evaporates outside of us.

When we are filled with stress or exhilaration, the flood of adrenaline permeates outside of us, and can be picked up by those around us. We feel each other's energetics and chemicals.

Our brain waves, be them delta, gamma, alpha or theta, can exude outside the brain. Theta is a calming brain wave, predominate in the state of trance or meditation. Theta waves, as they exude from an experienced meditator, can impact the brain waves of another person, facilitating the transition to a theta form. So, if there is ever a house for sale next to an ashram, buy it. You can save yourself a lot of meditation time by reaping the benefits of your neighbours' healing intentions.

By embracing the whole, we can positively affect our own health but also the health of those around us, the planet, our communities, the animals and the source of life itself. We are part of the dance called life. We affect it and it affects us.

So, the question becomes: how can our stress, anxiety and burnout be truly only about us, or even about our nervous system alone? Understanding the whole allows us to open to the possibility of exploring our relationships (to self and others), our environment, our social lives, our values, our nutrition, our circadian rhythms. Everything is on the table. Taking a broad and comprehensive look at all the aspects at play gives you the greatest opportunity to head in the direction of opening towards a fuller and more authentic experience of life.

Key points:

- Connection, reciprocity and mutuality are at the core of nature, including our innate nature.

- Energy is in constant flow and constantly interchanging.

- Life affects us, and we affect life.

chapter 9

YOUR INNER CRITIC

"You yourself, as much as anybody else in the entire universe, deserve your love and affection."

– Buddha

I was recently a participant in a personal development week where people came together to explore themselves deeply and take the time to look within courageously and gently. What I discovered about myself was profound.

One day began with a discussion on broadcasting: the concept that despite our best efforts to hide away our feelings from the world, people are very good at picking up signs. We 'broadcast' our feelings. The job in the group was to comment on what you had 'picked up' from each other through the previous few days. It was a chance to bravely own our stuff, and see what we reflect out to the world.

One man in our group, Richard, was a smartly dressed, fit man in his early 40s. He was active and often commented on how good he was feeling. He was always first up to speak and I felt he was having trouble being authentic. I felt like he was trying too hard, his effortful mind was blocking his ability to connect. It came around to my turn, and I shared this with him. He wasn't happy with my comments. My honesty had seemingly insulted Richard. When it came to his turn to speak about what he saw in me, he said one word. Resistant.

As the day went on, I started to feel ashamed. Perhaps I had said too much. It bothered me so much that I spoke with the lead facilitator the next morning. I told her that I felt that I had overstepped the boundary and felt like I needed to apologise. She reflected on the session and said she agreed with everything I had said. She asked me whether my "inner critic" was at play.

THE VOICE INSIDE

It's entirely natural to have an inner critic. In fact, we all have one, so you are not alone. The voice feels like mockery, shame, shut down or humiliation.

We all have inside us a picture of what an ideal person is. They may be calm, confident, assertive, popular and worthy of praise. The issue is that we want to be that ideal person all the time. When we fall short of that ideal, the inner critic steps in. It makes us feel guilty, chastises and berates us. The higher the internal ideal we set for ourselves the more ammunition the critic has to mock us and make us feel bad about ourselves.

The inner critic gets activated when we feel there is danger, or when we must toe the line or play small. It arrives when we feel vulnerable, fearful or overwhelmed. It feels like there is another person's voice trying to silence us, control us or intimidate us into a sense of submission. It can be so constant that over time we stop noticing it. When this happens, we may wind up believing the critical thoughts, which creates a deep sense of suffering.

The inner critic can make it seem necessary to adopt another persona: the cool girl, the arrogant intellect, the tough guy, the dominatrix, the sporty type. Sometimes we wear these masks so often and for so long that taking them off is terrifying. Sometimes it feels like we don't even know we are wearing a mask or even know the truth of ourselves.

THE VULNERABILITY UNDER THE CRITIQUE

We develop the inner critic around the age of three or four. Its internal voice can often sound remarkably like one or both of our parents or caregivers. Re-framing the self-critic as a source of internal protection can help you start to see it in a different light, and develop the skills to break down the irrational power it can have over your actions, feelings and sense of belonging.

Exercise: Inner Child

Try to visualise yourself as a scared, shy or timid child, at the age you were when the inner critic began to develop. At that age we don't have full use of language, intellect or autonomy.

Picture the inner critic as a voice that is trying to help you. By keeping you small, it is making sure you don't stand out in a crowd or do something daring, bold or something that offends someone else — because in the wilds, if a child did something bold or outlandish, they would have been at increased risk of being seen or hurt by a predator.

Consider writing about your inner child and inner critic in your Journal. What do they say? What tone do they use? Does this remind you of anyone you know? What do they look like?

It takes a lot of courage to face the painful aspects of our inner critic, especially if we have spent so long believing the negative critique they have fed us.

If we can practise turning towards ourselves in a kind way and recognising that this is in fact an inevitable part of human nature and a natural evolution of the brain, we can share the pain together and work towards befriending our internal protectors so that we can remain truer to who we are, rather than be shut down by ourselves inadvertently.

This requires a shift in willingness to look within, ownership of our biological and neurological tendencies and compassion towards ourselves and our need to learn a more productive way of being kind, true and supportive of ourselves.

THE ANTIDOTE

"With self-compassion, we give ourselves the same kindness and care we'd give to a good friend."

– Dr. Kristin Neff

One of the major fears we feel is when our sense of self is compromised; when we feel judged, rejected, abandoned or shunned. The reason this feels so intense is because we are social animals, and our survival is dependent on connection to each other. The antidote to a harsh self-critic is understanding the need for self-compassion, and practising it.

Dr Kristin Neff writes in her book *Self-Compassion: The Proven Power of Being Kind to Yourself*: "We confuse our thoughts and representations of ourselves for our actual selves, meaning that when our self-image is under siege, we react as if our very existence is threatened."

When this happens, our threat defence system uses four strategies to stay safe.

- **Fight:** We insult ourselves, by criticising, blaming, shaming, or belittling who we are.

- **Flight:** We feel anxious and irritated, we try to get away from this discomfort, using things such as food, alcohol, exercise, shopping or gambling to name a few.

- **Freeze:** We ruminate and obsess over our inadequacies and mistakes.

- **Submit:** We resign ourselves to the harsh criticisms and accept them as a part of the unworthiness that we are ashamed of.

This can leave us feeling highly anxious, depressed and angry with ourselves, others and the world. This can lead us to limit our relationships and our experiences in life. Acknowledging that the inner critic is not only a natural impact from childhood but one we all inherit can help us in sharing our humanness with others and allowing us to see it for what it is: a survival mechanism that we can choose to entertain or to reposition as a bit-player in our pursuit of aliveness.

The inner critic limits our aliveness. We continually harm ourselves when we chain ourselves inside this mental cage, and the saddest part is that we are trying to avoid the fear that is inside the cage too. We are running away in the same direction as from where it is coming.

To paraphrase a famous Einstein quote, we can't change anything with the same thinking that led to the issue in the first place. We need to look at the patterns, challenge what we think is true about ourselves and be brave enough to find the courage to share all our love with ourselves as well as those we hold dear. The trick is in learning the rules of our innate physiology and then consistently turning up for ourselves as equally deserving of compassion, care and love as anyone else.

Self-compassion is the act of sharing kindness with ourselves. It is offering ourselves a supportive voice, recognising that our feelings and experiences of life are valid. Self-compassion is also offered as protection of our boundaries; saying when you have had enough and allowing yourself limits. In Part 3, we will go through some self-compassion exercises to start the journey towards a safer internal environment and one reflective of our values of connection, love and belonging.

Exercise: Freedom Within

Take 15 minutes now to visualise or imagine what life would look like if you didn't have your current stress load.

You might like to imagine yourself in your favourite place, by a beach, in a forest or any place that makes you feel safe.

How would it feel, if you could quieten down your inner critic?

What would it feel like to not be held back by the criticism? What would you do differently?

Imagine joy arising inside of you. Can you imagine offering yourself the kindness you offer others?

Do you feel more peaceful or relaxed?

How would your body feel, if you were not burdened by the harshness of your inner critic?

Feel free to explore this via your imagination, or perhaps consider putting pen to paper. Whatever works for you.

LESSONS IN DISGUISE

"The most difficult times for many of us are the ones we give ourselves."

– Pema Chodron

Looking into the inner critic and seeing how it played out in my life allowed me to have one of the most profound shifts in self-awareness and self-worth that I have experienced in recent years. I backed myself and let Richard have the emotional response that he had had to my input. I continued to work on myself, knowing that what I shared was said with respect and great care.

One of the final exercises was to tell everyone in the group what we had received throughout the week-long process and what we saw in the others in our group. It was a beautiful exchange of compassion and sincerity.

Richard, who went first, said he had experienced an insightful week of new beginnings and more comfort with his emotions. When it was my turn to receive what the group had witnessed in me, Richard was the first to speak. "I just want to thank Michelle, on behalf of the group, for how much presence and effort she put into all of us, and into herself. She had a deep effect on me and I am so grateful," he said.

I was deeply touched by how much my own presence had supported someone, and how by simply turning up for myself, I inadvertently helped others to turn up for themselves. As we strive towards our authenticity and our courage, we in turn activate and inspire courage and sincerity in those around us.

We never know where our lessons will come from, and they are often wrapped in obscure disguises. By learning to better manage my inner critic, staying present and open and wanting to become the best version of myself, I paved the way for others to do the same. As social creatures we are bound by our energy, our biology, our chemistry and our wisdom.

Key Points:

- It is natural to have an inner critic. It develops in childhood and it is part of our survival neurology.

- The voice shuts you down and makes you feel bad about yourself, telling you that you are not good enough.

- Recognising and addressing the inner critic can make a profound difference to your mental health.

- Self-love and compassion are game-changers for those suffering chronic stress, anxiety and burnout.

part 2

EMBRACING THE WONDER WITHIN

chapter 10

BEYOND THE BEATING OF THE DRUM

"It's not what you look at that matters, it's what you see."

– Henry David Thoreau

In 1994, when I was in fourth-year medicine, I did my cardiology rotation. I remember sitting in a small tutorial room on the fifth floor of the Alfred Hospital, learning to read the electro-cardiogram (ECG). Aubrey Pitt, a renowned cardiologist, told us: "The heart is a pump, nothing more, nothing less." I sat there, feeling dejected and sad. It felt immediately wrong to call my inner core a simple pump. I intuitively sensed that my heart was so much more. Do you feel that too?

What I have since discovered about the science and the philosophy of the heart paints a very different picture to the professor's simple and primitive view. Yes, the heart is a vital pump, but it also holds our deepest mystery and connects us all together more strongly than any other part of the human body.

Poets, songwriters, lovers and storytellers have revered the essence of the heart for thousands of years, waxing lyrical about its magnificence. Rumi, a 15th century Sufi poet, wrote: "Your heart knows the way. Run in that direction." Carl Jung said "your vision will become clear only when you look into your heart," and in our modern era, Mary Oliver espoused that we should "keep some room in your heart for the unimaginable".

It is likely that you have, at least once in your life, received the advice to "follow your heart". We all intuitively know the difference between following our heads or following our hearts. But do we know how to do that? Could there be ways to actively get to know our heart's wisdom a little more closely, so that when that advice is needed, we have a way to tap into ourselves and find the way?

Our language holds hidden clues about the depth and integrity of the human heart. We collectively use terms such as kind hearted, whole hearted, brave hearted and cold hearted to indicate a person's depth and integrity. When we speak intimately, we call it a heart-to-heart. When we fall out of love, we know our heart feels broken.

This is not only in the domain of the West. It is found throughout many cultures. The Japanese character for "to listen" is made up of four different characters: one for the ear, one for the eyes, one for undivided attention and the other for the heart. The Chinese character for heart also means centre, core, feeling and thinking. The words for virtue, love, intention and listen all contain the character of the heart within them.

To Listen

Ear

You
Eyes
Undivided
Attention

Heart

When we feel deeply emotional, in both pleasant emotional states and those that are felt as unsettling, we often touch our hearts, holding them dearly. In many of the world's religions, the heart is seen as the "seat of the soul". The Babylonians, Mesopotamians and Ancient Greeks viewed the heart as the primary organ for decision making, emotions and morality.

OPENING UP TO THE HEART

"When our hearts are open and awake we care instinctively"

– Tara Brach

Traditional medical systems also reveal the significance of the heart's role in health. In traditional Chinese medicine the heart houses the 'shen', which roughly translates to the spirit. They say when the spirit is sick, the whole body is sick. The heart is seen as the governor to all other systems.

This is like the ancient Judaic system, where the heart centre is called the 'Tif Fer et'. This represents balance, harmony and beauty. In the Kabbalah, the heart is given the title of Central Sphere, the only core organ that touches all the others. This ancient metaphor is mirrored in our innate physiology.

It wasn't until I was four months into my training in traditional Vietnamese acupuncture, in Ho Chi Minh, that I realised that there had been no mention of the brain in all the 12 meridian pathways. In this system the brain is regarded as a machine, akin to a computer system, that requires input from the experiences, emotions and relationships of the body.

William Harvey (1578–1657), an English doctor who was influential in describing the circulatory system and how it delivers blood to the body and brain, is quoted as saying: "Every affection of the mind that is attended either with pain or pleasure, hope or fear, is the cause of an agitation whose influence extends to the heart." The heart feels it all and it is involved in all and therefore must become a key player in any plan to manage stress, anxiety or burnout.

This wisdom has been espoused for thousands of years by people who we as a culture revere, yet in a modern medical sense we still consider these sentiments to be "soft, mushy and somewhat weak". It seems modern Western culture is not interested in bringing the heart into our lives, work or health care. Medicine is delivered in the same patriarchal system that encourages boys to "harden up". Medical school was implicitly about becoming tough; being able to work long shifts of 14 hours or more and turning up the next day to do it all over again.

I remember going for a job interview once and chatting about my special interests in nutritional and mind-body medicine. The principal doctor of the clinic pulled a disgruntled face and told me they were "looking for someone to help them with real medicine".

We minimise the power of the emotions, the power of love, and belittle it as if it is secondary to our survival. But it is vital. We are at a point of change in this world, and people are waking up to the damaging effects of this disparaging attitude to emotional expression, vulnerability and connection.

Exercise: Reflect On Your Heart

Take a moment to reflect on these questions.

- How do you view your heart? Is it a mere pump? Or does it somehow hold your resonance? Does your heartbeat respond to your life?

- Is there something inside you that tells you your heart sits in your core?

- Is it where you love and care from? Is it where you sometimes feel from?

- Can you or do you let it guide you?

These are all good questions and there may not be clear answers, but if poets, lovers, song writers, artists, linguists, entire cultures and medical systems, psychiatrists, eminent Nobel prize-winning physicists and literary greats over thousands of years are to be believed, starting to consider your heart as a place of truth, safety and trust is an invitation worth considering.

If you are of the pump lineage, get curious about that belief. Everyone I have met and spoken to has inherently felt there is a sense of something special within our heart, an intelligence, a guidance. Is it mere metaphor, or could we actually use this essence to help guide us through this experience we call our lives? Could this be part of the opportunity that Hippocrates was referring to all those years ago?

Emotional intelligence (EQ) is a term coined by psychologists John Mayer and Peter Salovey. This definition broadened the role of intelligence to include the quality of our emotional relationships. There are five domains to EQ: knowing one's emotions, handling and managing one's emotions, motivating oneself, being tuned into the emotions of others and handling relationships. This awareness in both self and others is associated with greater successes in life in the areas of happiness and satisfying relationships. People with high EQ were found to be more flexible, more optimistic and stress resilient.

Key Points:

- The heart's qualities have been integral in the understanding of indigenous and traditional holistic healing systems.

- Poets, sages, and even languages speak of the inherent qualities of the heart: authenticity, compassion, kindness and courage.

- Our emotional lives impact every cell of our beings and shape our moments and our lives.

- Attending to the heart's virtues is associated with increased optimism, happiness and a sense of connection.

chapter 11

THE EMBRYOLOGY AND ANATOMY OF THE HEART

"There is a voice that doesn't use words. Listen."

– Rumi

We are a culture that is born from science. It permeates our medicine, our educational systems and our workplaces. Science provides the platform from which we evolve our thinking and understanding of the world and our place within it. I love science and I love the exploration, the details and the wonder that it brings. Using science as a way of understanding how we work, and all of the interconnections that we are naturally hooked into, helps us to understand our why in the universe. It provides the platform to help us find the meaning and purpose that we crave and need to reach the heights of our human potential.

Science gives us the permission to grow, it provides the foundation and security we need to open to new possibilities of thinking and doing in this life. Part 2 will teach you what you need to know to open to new understandings of the inner workings of the body. We have inside us one of the most fascinating and incredible systems in the known universe and most of us have no idea how we work. Learning about it can help us develop more gratitude, curiosity and confidence. This may support us on the journey to self-empowerment, self-compassion and peace.

Embryology isn't something we all know about, but it is a fascinating way of looking at how we have evolved over time. Taken as a whole, we are the custodians of the most biologically advanced living system in the known universe! Let's focus in on the heart.

- The heart is fully formed and beating when the embryo is only four weeks old.

- The first brain cell starts to form when the embryo is 12 weeks old.

- The heart is fully functioning, autonomous and beating before the brain is formed.

- It beats without input from the brain, a process known as auto-rhythm, but the brain controls the rate of the beating via the autonomic nervous system.

- The heart has its own independent nervous system.

- When a person has a heart transplant, the nerves that connect the heart to the new brain are not able to be reconnected. Therefore, the recipient has a new heart, which is beating via its own autorhythmic ability, but no connection to or from the recipient's brain.

- There is bi-directional communication between the heart and the brain. When the heart tells the brain what to do, it must follow the instruction, but when the brain tells the heart what to do, it has its own way of deciphering and discerning the message and deciding for itself what action will occur.

This last fact was discovered by physiologists Beatrice and John Lacey[8]. They found that when the brain sent messages to the heart, the heart didn't automatically follow them. Rather, the heart seemed to respond according to a more comprehensive distinctive logic. For example, when the brain sent a signal of arousal to the heart and the body, sometimes the heart rate would go up alongside the body, and other times it would do the opposite. The outcome of the signalling by the brain seemed to depend on the issue at hand.

And yes, that heart of yours is one hell of a pump. It beats about 100,000 times per day — that is 40 million beats per year and more than three billion beats per lifetime. It will beat unrelentingly for you for an average lifespan of 84 years. It pumps about seven litres of blood per minute around a system that covers about 95,000 kilometres (approximately two times the Earth's circumference!)

THE WAY THE HEART COMMUNICATES

"The quieter you are able to become, the more you are able to hear."

– Rumi

One role of the heart is to make sure the blood is pumped through the cardiovascular system and that every cell in the human body receives information stored within the blood. This includes nutrients and water from the digestive system, inflammatory and immune cells from the immune system, hormonal and chemical messengers from the brain and endocrine system, cholesterol that is produced in the liver to help maintain the integrity of the cell membrane and oxygen from the lungs to give the cells what they need to produce energy. It then takes all the cell's toxic waste products away. So, the heart has connection with every cell in the body.

This pump is more than a simple 'squeeze and relax' effect. It has a way to direct and align the blood flow to the various organs in response to the needs of the body, using emotional, intuitive and physical requirements. It is the main driver of harmony between the systems in the body.

There are four different ways the heart communicates with the rest of the cells in the body.

1. Neurologically (the heart-brain)

Think of this like a little brain inside the heart, with sufficiently sophisticated networks that allow it to behave independently to the brain inside the head.

Dr John Armour from Halifax University has found evidence that the heart-brain, as the researchers named it, can think, feel, sense, learn and remember. Via its neural tissues, the heart assesses its pressure, rate, hormonal and neurochemical messages and flow. It translates that to information which then travels up via the vagus nerve to the primitive part of the brain called the medulla. The medulla is primarily involved in the regulation of the autonomic nervous system (which we will learn more about in the next chapter). The autonomic nervous system has a regulating effect on the whole body. But the nerve messages go beyond the medulla and travel up into the limbic system (emotions and memory, and endocrine control centre) and then onto the cortical areas of the body, responsible for critical thinking, forward judgement, cognition and consciousness.

The heart's input into these areas can be either stimulating or inhibiting. This is thought to be the pathway that helps us modify and potentiate our learning, our emotional regulation and performance.

The thalamus is part of the limbic system responsible for sensory perception, consciousness and wakefulness. It is a hub-like area of the brain which receives impulses from the entire body, and then transfers these to various parts of the brain for processing. In the 1980s German scientists found the pathway from the heart to the thalamus and found that the heart played a role in the overall synchronisation of all cortical activity, thereby affecting cognitive performance and activity[9].

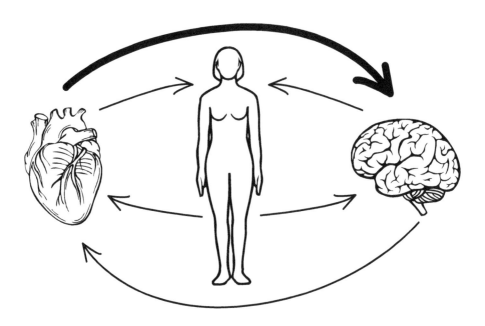

There is more neural information flowing from the heart to the brain as compared to the other way around. The heart uses a multitude of ways to decipher and interpret information from the environment and the body. The coherence of the flow of information sent to the brain via the heart has implications on the optimal functioning of the brain.

This throws new light on the wisdom from the ancients, that listening closely to the body and the heart can help us review how we perceive the world, and therefore quite simply change our reality. This is vitally important in the case of stress, anxiety and burnout, where often our reality appears so oppressive and out of balance. Listening closely to the heart and the body can start to establish the pathways needed for transformation and new understandings.

2. The pulse wave (rhythmic beating patterns)

If we go back to quantum physics, you will recall that energy moves in wave forms. The wave forms that are centralised by the heart's information are more than the standardised pressure of a simple pump. These wave forms, or rhythmic patterns, travel faster than the blood. The rhythm creates a resonance that can be read by the autonomic nervous system, the blood vessels, the endocrine glands and the breath. The heart has a language, so every cell in the body has a way of listening and responding to its rhythm.

The time intervals that naturally occur between the beats of our heart are known as heart rate variability (HRV). The more variability in our heart rate, the better. HRV is an easy way to see how our emotional states are reflected in our heart's rhythms.

When the body is in an uncomfortable emotional state such as anger, fear, blame or insecurity, the heart rhythm goes into a jagged and disordered pattern. Positive feelings such as love, compassion, forgiveness and appreciation have been matched to a more harmonious rhythm that is balanced, and smooth. This is called internal coherence.

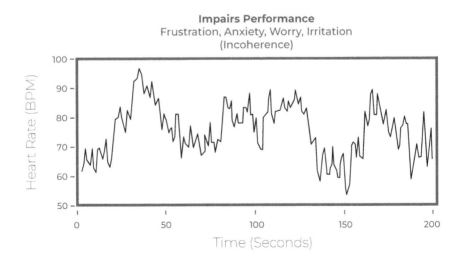

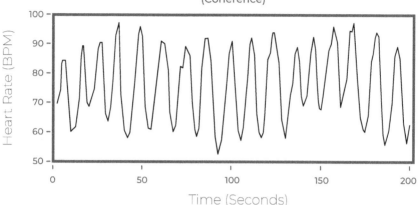

Promotes Optimal Performance
Positive Emotions, Appreciation, Love, Care
(Coherence)

Heart rate variability is the beat-to-beat variation. It changes and adapts depending on the attitudes, emotions and sensations inside the body. When the body is in a state of agitation, frustration and irritation the heart beat is less variable and more incoherent. When the person returns or manifests a state of peacefulness, gratitude or compassion, the heart rate variability increases. The heart beat becomes more coherent and in rhythmic flow.

The greater the coherence the better the information is processed by the brain. This is associated with greater productivity, creativity, and learning.

Image and research credit: HeartMath Institute

When a system is said to be in coherence, it is a system experiencing maximal power and efficiency, where virtually no energy is wasted. Coherency is the ultimate goal for heightened productivity and personal development.

Research from the HeartMath Institute has shown that when we are in a feeling state such as love, compassion, care and appreciation, it improves the coherence of the heart. It enhances our cognition, creativity, learning, problem solving skills and emotional decision making, creates a sense of inner peace and calm, and decreases the impact of stress and anxiety on the body.

The heart is our internal coherency governor and a major player in our return to health and wellbeing. There are many tools to cultivate coherence, which we will explore in this book. Appreciation is the first thing that I recommend you try to generate. Even if we are in crisis, we can usually sit back and appreciate *something*, be it the smell of freshly mowed grass, the sunshine on our back, a lovely vista or image or a kind gesture from a friend. For some people it can be difficult in a state of fear, extreme stress to conjure up feeling of love and compassion, as anger, resentment and grief can get in the way, but appreciation seems in the playing field for most of us to try.

Exercise: Cultivate Coherence Through Appreciation

Sit comfortably on your chair or lie still in your bed. Set a timer for five minutes. Take a long slow deep breath and tell yourself: "There is nothing more important to do at this time and nowhere else I need to be."

As your breath steadies, even just a little, bring in a moment, image, person, pet or event that you can appreciate. Try to bring the feeling into your heart space. And as you focus on the sense, breathe into your heart space and try to let the breath make the feeling of appreciation grow, as if your heart is now filled with appreciation. Really focus on the feeling in your heart, and see if you can tap into the pleasure it is giving you. Stay with it, until the buzzer goes off.

It is great to recognise how quickly we can change our internal automated systems through our connection to our breath.

3. Electromagnetic energy

The electro-cardiogram (ECG) is a common test, ordered by doctors millions of times a day across the world. Ten wires are stuck to certain points of the skin to pick up the heart's electromagnetic energy patterns, to diagnose things like heart attacks and arrhythmias.

The heart generates the strongest electromagnetic field (EMF) of the body — it is 5,000 times stronger than the EMF produced by the brain. The heart's field permeates every cell of the body, but it also radiates out beyond the skin. This field can be detected by machines called magnetometers up to three meters away. It is thought the machine is the limiting factor, and that if we had more sensitive machines, we would find the field radiates out further afield — perhaps indefinitely. This gives new understanding to what the ancient shamans talked about, that one person's heart can impact another's far away.

Have you ever walked into a room and everyone falls silent, and you realise that you have just walked in on an argument? You haven't heard any words or seen any violence, but you can feel the energy in the room. You just walked into these people's heart spaces, and you have picked up the jagged energy exuding out of their bodies. We live in each other's heart spaces. We influence each other without words and without actions. We have so much responsibility to look after our heart's energy, which will transform the energy in others, near and possibly even further afield.

Exercise: Your Heart's Energy

Take a moment to place your hand on your heart. See if you can feel this energy by touching your skin.

Take a moment to send some loving thoughts to your heart, even if it feels a little strange to do so. This amazing heart of yours has been beating since you were an embryo. Take this moment to connect to it, to its wonder, to its magnificence.

It communicates with every cell, it impacts you inside and out, you can physically send appreciative thoughts to those you love. Tap into this opportunity to transform the lives of others. Feel the sincerity of attempting to bring goodness to another person.

4. Bio-chemically (hormones and neurotransmitters)

This mode of communication provides a new way of recognising the complex, intricate and whole system approach the body has in maintaining its integrity and balance. Hormones are chemical messages made by a gland. The message travels from the gland to other parts of the body to influence another system. You might be familiar with hormones such as oestrogen, insulin and cortisol.

In the early 1980s the heart was reclassified to an endocrine organ, when it was discovered that it produces a hormone called atrial natriuretic factor (ANF), which regulates blood pressure, body fluid and electrolyte balance. On further research it was found that ANF can inhibit the release of cortisol, and influence the growth and function of the reproductive organs. It amazingly influences the immune system and is associated with more motivated behaviours.

Neurochemicals are chemical compounds that influence the activity of the brain. Some common ones you might know of are serotonin and dopamine. The heart produces these chemicals as well as the brain. These chemicals influence how we feel, what motivates us and how we behave.

More research is needed to fully understand how this complex soup of chemicals, neural information and pathways work, but it is irrefutable that the heart is much more than a simple pump. Acknowledging this opens up a whole new opportunity to explore our intimate and personal relationship to this vital organ inside our chests.

Key Points:

- The heart and the brain communicate in a bi-directional manner.
- The heart communicates via its rhythmic energy patterns, its electromagnetic field, its blood flow and its hormonal/neurochemical pathways.

- The heart was fully formed and fully functional eight weeks prior to the first brain cell being formed.

- The energetic heart space extends beyond the body. It is a part of how we exchange and receive energy.

chapter 12

MY HEART'S STORY

"To heal, you have to go to the root of the wound and kiss it all the way up."

– Rupi Kaur

I have suffered from anxiety, stress and burnout. Despite having the knowledge of mind-body medicine, life got in my way, and I got in life's way. I was certainly not in harmony with my body's wisdom. During some of the darkest times, I sensed very strongly that I would get very sick if I continued the way I was going.

Dr Jill Bolte is an American neurologist and author of the book *My Stroke of Insight — a Brain Scientist's Personal Journey*. In 1996 Jill woke up with a throbbing headache. Ignoring the severity of it, she jumped on her exercise machine. A few minutes later she noticed a strange feeling in her left hand. It appeared to her as a claw. In fact, her whole body felt odd and not her own. Jill was experiencing a massive stroke, a haemorrhage inside the right hemisphere of her brain. Because of her intimate knowledge of the brain, she realised she needed help but she also felt this overwhelming sense of fascination at witnessing her own demise from the inside out.

She woke up in the hospital bed after surgery feeling expansive and enormous, like she was in connection with the whole universe. She recalls thinking, "how am I ever going to squeeze the enormousness of myself back inside this tiny body?" But her recovery was not instant nor quick. Despite her knowing that the brain can grow new neurons and make new connections, it took her eight years to recover from the damage to her brain.

The right hemisphere of the brain is where we hold the ability to see expansively, to feel the wholeness in the universe and acknowledge consciousness in its purest form, whereas the left hemisphere is involved in data, names, numeracy and language. The right looks at the big picture, the left looks at the details. The left brain identifies the individual, the right is the relationship to the whole. They are balanced by the input from the body. They balance each other. As Jill recovered, she became even more interested in the workings of the brain. In chatting to those who had the opposite side affected, she found they experienced a completely different experience to her. Those with a left hemisphere defect reported feeling obsessed by details, unable to let errors in language fall by the wayside, and they felt critical of everything. They felt disconnected from the whole and unable to experience a sense of expansiveness that Jill had.

My burnout experience felt like that. I had to talk myself into getting out of bed every day. When I arrived at work, I had to massage my jaw muscles and practise saying "hello" to the staff in the car before I walked in. I was empty, stressed, miserable and confused. I had lost my empathy and I was scared I wouldn't get it back.

I was doing all the right things — meditating, yoga, walking daily, sleeping well, eating well and looking after myself — but there was nothing I could do on a physical or cognitive level that could help. I was trying too hard, hoping to receive 'signs from the universe' to guide me — an arrow and words saying, "hey Michelle, go this way!"

My heart was crying. Eventually I realised I had to let it lead the way on this journey. But I had dug my hole so deep that getting out was a mammoth task.

Shutting the doors of a general practice has unforeseen implications. You must keep access to all medical records for up to 21 years. You need to make every attempt to inform the patients and make sure you have handover of all 10,000 of them — not to mention the staff payouts, redundancies and upsetting the livelihoods of 18 people. So, I was in a situation where it was stressful to close and stressful to stay open.

Knowing the science of my heart and the wisdom that I had within me, my only choice was to trust.

THE WISDOM OF THE HEART

The language of the heart is subtle, poetic and somewhat excruciatingly puzzling. It uses pulse waves, energy and internal messages to weave its magic in our lives. Deep within, my heart had been speaking, but the life I was living was noisy and full and I couldn't hear its whispers, even though I knew they were there.

The way the heart shares its wisdom can be quite mysterious. As I was going through the process of working out the best way to proceed, I attended a regular monthly meditation group.

Every month as we sat down in the room, the facilitator would put two oracle cards underneath our cushions. Halfway through the evening we would have an opportunity to look at them and see if they might help us through a symbol or meaning that could shift our clarity. There was always the option of putting the card back and re-choosing if you felt that the card didn't suit you.

I was going through the process of making the tough decision to sell my business. In the previous months I had picked up cards with words such as resilience, non-judgement, determination. With these cards in hand, I felt akin and connected. These words reflected back to me my process, and how I was digging deep inside myself for courage and strength.

One evening, I overturned my card and the word I got was joy. My initial instinct was to put it back and pick again. I sat with it for a while, but I couldn't feel the resonance. It felt frivolous, insipid and weak. It didn't have the grunt of resilience, or the sense of striving like determination did. I kept it by my cushion. I tried to be patient and trust it, but I wasn't feeling it.

A niggly feeling stayed with me throughout the following week. Why was it that I felt the urge to hand back joy? And then it came to me. I realised I didn't "do joy". I fleetingly experience it, I encourage others to find it, but I didn't run headlong into it. I was addicted to hard, to challenge, to striving, to achieving, and I had forgotten the sweetness of life, the simple pleasure of joy. What a revelation. I didn't do joy!

This is how the heart shares it gifts. It doesn't have the dedicated pathways of language to reveal itself, so it operates in a more cryptic way. Knowing that the heart loves to be in joy, I understood that this was a message from a deeper part of me; this was an opportunity to open to joy, to seek it, to savour it, to honour it.

This new awareness was a profound shift. It was the invitation into my aliveness. Joy is deeply connected with aliveness. Making this a valid way to spend time — nothing else to gain except the very experience of joy itself — was a miracle message that I now honour, respect and admire.

ON THE OTHER SIDE OF BURNOUT

The road out of burnout was way longer than I thought it would be. In the early days after the sale of my clinic, I had expected my anger and grief to subside as a new life unfolded. Instead, it got worse.

The anger was intense. Mostly I was angry at how hard it was. I could see my brain, which was used to being constantly 'on', trying to remain in that state. Stress was familiar and in some weird way felt comfortable. Strategising, planning, striving, pushing: that had been my normal for so long that my nervous system had become automated.

Luckily, I had good counsel, outside myself and also within. Even though my body and brain weren't resting as planned, I used my heart to know that is what was needed. I had to fight the inclination to jump straight back on the horse. If I wanted to transform my life, I had to fully close the chapter of the last one. When someone we are close to dies, we don't immediately go on with our lives. We stop, we process, we remember, we learn. We take the time to re-evaluate, re-establish a new normal and we acquiesce into a new way. This needed to be the same.

The heart holds the ingredient needed to maintain the integrity of a change. It can hold the intention needed, even if that intention is ill conceived, or is tiny and intangible. Listening to the body is a skill worthy of every ounce of our lives, especially when we are suffering from stress, anxiety and burnout. We need to fight for ourselves.

My automated brain was getting in the way of my recovery and I am grateful that I knew how to recognise it. But it wasn't easy. The heart does speak to us, but it is shy. It is always on our side. It will never betray us, nor ever lead us astray. But its messages don't always make immediate sense, or seem rational or practical.

The journey to the heart is difficult at the beginning, but it is a skill we can learn and must learn if we are truly going to navigate our way out of anxiety, stress and burnout. If we let our brains lead our lives, we are at the whim of entering into that world again and repeating the patterns of behaviour that caused the issues in the first place.

Since leaving the business, and starting a new life, despite the fear of a change in income and fear of failing as I pursue a dream such as writing this book, I feel comfortable in the new sense of aliveness that has come, in the slowing down and the seeing more, in the laughter that is palpable and joyous, in the new dreams that are alive.

We only get one chance at life and we can't turn back the clock of the years. I am proud of myself, for saving myself from the seductive illusion of the rat race. I am at the beginning of a whole new life, with a chance for freedom and wholeness, vitality and wonder. A life where my heart can speak and I now know how to listen.

Taking the time to explore whatever comes, in whatever way it comes, is the subtle way of opening to the inner wisdom that resides in us all. For me it was a small word on a card in the middle of a circle. Joy stirred me up, confused me and challenged my old patterns. It was only because I let it in, didn't dismiss it, and challenged myself to look at my reaction that I was able to see something that I didn't even know I needed to look at.

The heart has a special kind of wisdom, away from intellect, rational thought or reduction. Listening is the key that opens its door. You don't need to trust me — you just need to trust yourself, your stress, your anxiety and whatever situation you are in. There is gold in 'dem hills, and all you need to do is listen for it.

Key Points:

- Trust is essential to the journey of the heart.

- The heart speaks in elusive ways, it often waits for silence before it expresses itself.

- The normalisation of stress and the automation of the lower brain functions take over when we fall into old habits.

- Listening and sensing are critical skills to develop.

chapter 13

THE ROLE OF THE MIND

"Taking responsibility for one's own mind can lead to liberation of the self, and to the ability to offer nurturance and love to the next generation."

– Dr Daniel Seigel

What is the mind? Philosophers, poets, writers, doctors and psychologists have been exploring this question for thousands of years. Most of us feel like we know what it is for the purpose of everyday conversation. In the realm of science, it remains an illusive concept but one which is vitally important in learning how it relates to our emotional wellbeing.

Understanding the mind can help us use the holistic principles in this book to fundamentally challenge outdated approaches to stress, anxiety and burnout, and strengthen a transformative new approach that leans into our emotions.

The mind is often seen as residing in the brain, but this is not entirely accurate. It has four facets that scientists and deep thinkers can agree upon.

1. It is an information processing system, just like inside a computer. Information can be seen as energy flow, and the mind is an energy flow system. This alone may give us some clues that the heart may play a role in the construct of the mind, as the heart is the key modulator of our energetic messaging system throughout the body.

2. Sentient consciousness. Put simply, this is our ability to see what we are seeing. There are no other mammals on the planet, apart from the higher apes, that share this ability. Other animals and plants are said to have consciousness but without the sentience. This is the gift we have in this lifetime. It is a profound and influential aspect of the human journey and not to be disregarded.

3. Subjectivity. This is our ability to sense a feeling, to feel what we are feeling. This provides the uniqueness to our mindset and is how one person can feel something differently to another person in the same situation. This aspect of subjectivity defines our autonomy and individuality and allows us the governance to find our own way 'home'. As the saying goes, "one man's meat is another man's poison".

4. The fourth facet of the mind is that it is "emergent". It is a self-organising system, therefore it can create its own path and it can evolve. It is more than its parts, and by its nature it cannot be reduced to its parts. Your mind is whole and can never not be whole.

These principles of the mind are that of perception, adaptability, growth and flow. Our mind is thought to occupy the energetic space that lies in between our relationships. Our minds assist us in our relationships to others, to life and to change. We all by nature of our humanity can change our minds, to allow them to be more helpful, broader, open and receptive. These skills are not for the chosen one, they are within us all. By understanding the innate aspects of our humanness, we can own it, witness it and therefore make any adjustments that can help us to review what no longer serves us and work towards a better way of relating to the world, a way that can serve us better and go beyond surviving to thriving.

MINDFULNESS AND MINDLESSNESS

"In any given moment we are either practising mindfulness or we are practising mindlessness."

– Jon Kabat Zinn

Over the past decade the world has exploded with mindfulness-based courses, books and podcasts, and the word has become commonplace in the everyday language of our lives. We try to be mindful of others and ourselves, are encouraged to be mindfully body aware when doing the dishes, cutting carrots or speaking in a meeting, and are told to eat mindfully. It is being taught in kindergarten, schools, workplaces and even football clubs.

Mindfulness has incredible value in optimising our emotional, mental and physical health, but do we truly understand what it means to be mindful? I often find it interesting to approach such a complex concept by looking at its opposing view, to see if that can deepen our understanding. So, to understand mindfulness, let us ask ourselves: what does it mean to be mindless?

There are four aspects to the state of mindlessness.

1. When information and energy does not flow smoothly or in a coherent way. There is confusion or stagnation, doubt or fear. It is likely we all have a fair idea of what this feels like, when our chosen task feels awkward or ill-considered, and we end up agitated and frustrated. Many scholars, creatives, spiritual teachers and performance coaches will speak of the concept of flow. This was first coined by scientist Mihaly Csikszentmihalyi to describe the ideal state of coherence, creativity, joy and productivity. It is what runners call the zone, artists call the flow, meditators call the bliss. Anything else has elements of mindlessness attached.

2. An un-awareness of the lived experience of the self, and of life. When I was in a state of significant burnout, I would often arrive home from work having no clear recollection of the road I just travelled. I think this state is more common than most of us like to admit. I recall a time when one of my patients was diagnosed with a potentially terminal illness, and stated: "How could this happen? I haven't even lived." She was 73 years old.

    These are the people who for multiple reasons have followed a set path, never straying or finding their own way, whether because of conditioning, fear, martyrdom or simply a missed opportunity. They were too fearful to take hold of this exquisite risk we call life. They lived a safe life, protected from even the consciousness of their own lived experience. This is a state of semi-unconsciousness. Sometimes second chances just simply don't come along. Did we really sign up for this?

3. A lack of understanding of the feelings at play, either via denial, ignorance, delusion or inexperience. When we are operating in a mindless paradigm, we are not in connection with our unique and personal way of interpreting the world around us — our likes, dislikes, yearning, disgust and everything in between. We question how we feel, rely on others to help us understand the way we feel, and are out of touch with our feelings and our inner desires. Mindlessness is a state of not knowing how we feel or not allowing ourselves to feel what we are feeling.

4. Mindlessness is also a state of non-emergence. It lacks an internal self-organisation. There is a scatteredness to this aspect, a confusion and lack of ownership of the relationship we have with life. Because of this the person is in a state of stagnation and potentially at risk of devolving rather than evolving.

Take a minute to absorb the breadth and depth of the state of mindlessness.

Mindfulness, on the other hand, is a state of being that remains attentive to the moment-by-moment awareness of either our thinking or feeling, and/or bodily sensations, including our senses of hearing, smelling, seeing, touching, tasting or spatial awareness.

Mindfulness also involves both non-judgement, curiosity and awareness. It is an attention exercise which aims to develop our ability to live life with our full human faculties rather than react with re-hashed and automated responses.

Learning, embracing and celebrating the state of mindfulness will help you connect to your uniqueness, your creativity, your potential, and the very experience of life itself.

You have an opportunity now to truly embrace this life you have, with all its stress, drama, pain and suffering, all your regrets, misgivings and mistakes, all your everything! Take this opportunity to truly take on the practise of mindful aliveness.

Mindfulness is a practise that supports us:

- In our lived experience, by helping us explore and engage with our felt sense.

- In opening up to the consciousness that we all have.

- By giving us an opportunity to allow our energy to flow, so that the information we are receiving is flowing as it is, and we have a spaciousness to receive it as we receive it.

- To evolve facets of the mind and support its emergent and self-organising qualities. This by its nature means it can support its own becoming.

Wow! Isn't that a practise we might feel inspired to do every day? I'm setting you a challenge to do this next exercise every day for the next week. It only need be five minutes a day and it is better to do it daily for a shorter time than weekly for a longer time. Your job is to see what comes. Remember you are building muscle in awareness, self-respect, listening and being real. Nothing is off the cards.

Exercise: Inward Explorer

Set a five-minute timer. Take a moment to practise being present with whatever you are feeling right now, without distractions. You may be hungry, tense, angry. You might feel flat, humiliated, unworthy. You might have a knot in your tummy, a lump in your throat and tightness across the chest. You may be feeling grateful, warm, joyful or perhaps even neutral. You might feel confused, you might feel numb or you may even be feeling nothing at all. Can you sit with yourself?

Take a few long, slow, deep breaths. Notice the breath exactly how it is. Is it tight, irregular, scrappy? Can you watch it coming into rhythm? Deepen it, lengthen it and see if you can support it coming into flow.

Try not to judge yourself for the way you feel, just feel it as it is. Even if it is making you feel more uncomfortable, try to stay with it. Try to become a witness for your body to express itself. Remember that stress, anxiety and burnout are real experiences, trying to be felt.

Just breathe. Notice how you feel. Do this until the buzzer goes.

If you feel a little overwhelmed by this, try one minute. You can stop anytime but try to do it consistently every day.

If you feel any fear rising during mindfulness exercises, see if you can hold it a little longer. Try to be curious. Recognise that it isn't pleasant, but know that it won't harm you. Feeling fear is something none of us find pleasant, but by feeling it we can allow it room to move. Try labelling it as fear, saying things such as "this is my fear", "I'm feeling my anxiety", "this is what fear feels like, it isn't pleasant but it can't hurt me".

Keep breathing through it.
Breathe.

Mindfulness strengthens our inner explorer. The more you stay, the more you will learn.

Key Points:

- The mind is made of four facets: subjectivity, information flow, awareness and growth.

- Listening for and sensing our own personal interpretation of life is essential to the growth of the mind.

- The process of self-inquiry is essential for the development of mindfulness and vice versa.

- Practising these skills helps you refine them, enjoy them and maximise the learnings that come from them.

chapter 14

THE BRAIN AND THE WHOLE

"Inviting our thoughts and feelings into awareness allows us to learn from them rather than be driven by them."

– Dr Daniel Seigel

Our brains are magnificent machinists who love a good story. What I mean is that we have evolved to listen to story, to learn through story and to understand our own worldview through stringing together the patterns of these stories.

This is not only because we are all artists and poets. It is a way that we connect, but it also allows for efficiency in our brains. If we can take a small amount of information and run it into the song lines of our past experiences, we can save a lot of time and energy. We don't need to listen to long-winded stories; we simply take a similar pathway and head to the destination nice and quickly.

This is the power of automation. Anyone in business today can espouse the need for automation, an energy efficient process that hands over an action to an automatic system. Our brain is masterful at automation. We all can recall the intense focus we needed when we first turned the ignition key in our first ever driving lesson. The focus to re-adjust the mirrors, put our seatbelt on, check the petrol, the steering wheel, the road, the oncoming cars and more. Our eyes constantly scanning, our brains firing for total focus, as we gently backed out of the driveway. Months later and the whole process becomes completely easeful.

The brain uses 25 per cent of our total glucose levels daily, despite being only two per cent of our total body weight. It is a hungry machine, so wherever it can, it will aim for automation for energy efficiency.

But we are at risk of automating our emotional responses, thoughts and feelings too. The more we respond in a certain way, the more likely we will respond the same way the following day. This is where we can run into trouble. We can become addicted to feeling guilty, addicted to our suffering, doubting ourselves and our choices, or getting angry with a driver when they don't indicate for long enough. If we don't become diligent and aware of these behaviours and thoughts, we get stuck in an automated pattern of life that may be okay, but may not be of our choosing, if you know what I mean.

Understanding that our brains run on auto most of the time is really important. When we are in a state of stress, anxiety or burnout, our brains are in survival mode. Survival mode is where we are trying to conserve energy as much as possible in order to defend ourselves against threat. We become hypervigilant and hyper-aware of potential attack. One of the best ways to create efficiency is to automate the way we perceive the world. Most of us think we are fully in control of what we think and what we believe is to be true. But by understanding the seductive nature of our brain's auto-pilot propensity and the fact we use this preferential energy saving mode whenever we can, we can see that most of us go through life pre-filling our stories and reiterating the same view of life over and over. Discovering automation and its limitations to our ability to change our thinking opens our minds and transforms our perspective, so we can find the understanding we need to persist through the challenges. This can be totally transformational. It takes courage and kindness to look within, to see our automation for what it is and challenge ourselves to look a little longer, listen a little harder, ask more questions, be a little more understanding and try to see things in a different way.

FUN BRAINY FACTS

The human brain is touted to be the most complex biological system known in the universe.

- Your brain weighs about two kilograms, contains about 1.1 trillion cells and 100 billion neurons. Each neuron contains about 5,000 different connections. The permutations of all this are more infinite than there are stars within the universe.

- The brain is said to be plastic — this means it changes with experiences, thoughts, exercise and memories. We can heal our nervous system like we can heal our skin, it just takes a little more persistence, practise, repetition, and know how.

- Our brain and nervous system can be tuned into safety or tuned into danger.

- The brain uses electrical impulses, neuro-chemicals and neuro-hormones to communicate.

- It is made up of mostly fat, protein and water, and uses glucose for energy.

- The brain requires more energy to sleep than resting on the couch.

- As you read this literally trillions of chemical signals have gone off inside your head.

THE EVOLUTIONARY BRAIN

Your brain has evolved and is still evolving. Human evolution has arisen from single cell origins, through to bacteria, jellyfish, amphibians, reptiles, mammals, primates and into conscious humans. We still operate with these 'primitive' reflexes. For example when we taste something bad, we all screw up our faces in disgust, or when we are scared, our startle reflex kicks in... our heart rates go up along with our breath, and our muscles get tense, ready to run or attack. Evolution is like a renovation as opposed to a new build — you are left with many features you would perhaps like to change, but that would be too expensive and difficult.

There are three broad parts of the evolutionary brain.

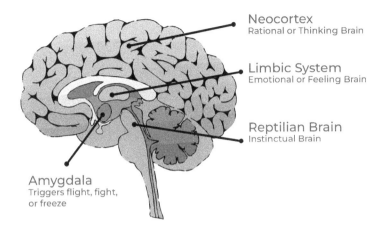

The human brain evolved over hundreds of thousands of years. The reptilian brain is also called the brain stem. As the human brain evolved over time, higher cortical structures were formed. The Limbic system is also called the mammalian brain or emotional brain, it includes the amygdala. The neo-cortex (also called the cortex) houses the pre-frontal cortex, this is also called the frontal lobe. This is the newest part of the brain in evolutionary terms.

1. The brain stem

The brain stem is often referred to as the reptilian system. It is emotionless, fast, automated and simplistic. Think of a crocodile on a riverbank. It does not feel guilt, remorse or anger. Its survival is not based on nurturing, it is based on well adapted instinct, armour, teeth and strength. The brain stem is the part of the brain that is focused solely on survival. It is responsible for our instinctual behaviour and we have no control over how it responds at all. The brain stem regulates our breath rate, our heart rate and blood pressure. It also plays a role in our interpretation of our senses, and it houses our vomiting reflex, posture responses and consciousness. If we are ever in the situation where we activate the sympathetic nervous system and we can neither fight or flee the situation, the brain stem can collapse us in order to survive — meaning we may faint or freeze if it deems necessary for survival.

2. The limbic system

This part of the brain is also called the mammalian part, or emotional brain. It evolved after the primitive brain and is thought to be in response to the need to survive the dinosaurs. Smaller mammals needed to think together to coordinate efforts to save themselves. Our evolutionary ancestors needed to be able to process emotions and memories quickly and develop a central and coordinated hub for this to occur. While a crocodile works alone, a pack of wolves band together, strategically supporting each other because of the group mentality.

Mastering social niceties, as we all know, requires a lot of effort and therefore a lot of brain power. So, the primary role of the limbic system is emotional reactivity, memory, perception and wakefulness regulation.

The limbic system houses the amygdala, the thalamus and the hippocampus. These parts of the brain think fast, react based on memory and if dominant, facilitate the emotional automation of our lives. For example, it is this part of the brain that gets a fright when we see a stick on the path, instantly think it is a snake, and jump away in response. It is the cortex that has the slower ability to decipher the automated response and choose to respond differently if required — for example, when you realise a few seconds later that the stick is just a stick, and calmly step over it.

3. The cortex

This is the most evolutionarily new part of the brain. It grew rapidly after the discovery of fire, cooking and an increased consumption of readily accessible foods such as meat. As our brains evolved and got bigger, this growth helped us become more socially connected and intelligent, and gave us the ability to plan, critically assess situations, be more discerning, and adapt to the external and internal environment.

It includes the frontal lobe for planning and critical thinking, the temporal lobe for listening and understanding, the parietal lobe for sensing, proprioception (our ability to know where we are in space) and language and the occipital lobe for vision.

All parts of the brain are in bi-directional communication with each other, but by dividing them into these three major areas, we can see why we tend to automate first before turning to our critical thinking skills.

By understanding this, we can see our reactivity as a matter of evolutionary history and biology rather than a flaw of our personality. We all share this commonality, and therefore all share the ability to transform this into new skills.

THE LIMBIC SYSTEM IN DEPTH

Now let's go a little bit deeper and explore more about the limbic system, its relationship to the frontal lobe and how it all connects. Hang in there, this is super important.

There are three parts to the limbic system: the amygdala, the hippocampus and the thalamus.

The Limbic System

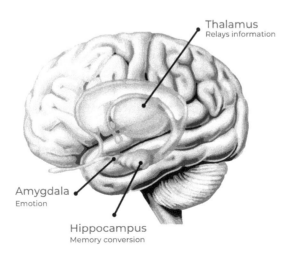

The limbic system is also called the mammalian brain or emotional brain. It is where we process our emotions, store memories and interpret our perceptions. The reflexive nature of the limbic system helps us to access our emotions quickly to respond to threat or danger.

The amgydala

This little almond-shaped part of the brain is called its alarm centre. Its role is to alert us to danger, instantly and quickly. You will have felt the effect of the amygdala if you have felt triggered by a snake slithering across the walking track, a challenging or embarrassing story inside your head, or something someone just said which reminded you of a painful or uncomfortable issue.

As we evolved, we needed a quick way to access memory so we could automatically protect ourselves from danger. Imagine you are a baby monkey, growing up in the forests, and your mother tells you about these big stripy animals with huge teeth called tigers. With drama in her voice, she speaks of the potential danger you would be in if you came face to face with a tiger. This makes you feel scared, and that fear heightens your ability to lay down those negative memories, so that you can access them without second guessing yourself. A few weeks later when you are off playing and you see a glimmer of orange, you scamper up the tree to safety, without a second thought. If you didn't have that skill, you would instead have to spend time recalling what your mother said about tigers. Perhaps those extra few seconds of deliberation might mean you are now a dead monkey.

This alarm system has evolved to quickly react to danger, and to help us seek protection. The problem arises when it is overactive because of chronic stress or enlarged because of a constant feeling of threat in our lives. Modern life doesn't have tigers roaming the street, but we do have financial stress, long working hours, rude and narcissistic bosses or aggressive partners. For many people their amygdala is larger than it ideally should be, and therefore it is getting triggered at even the slightest look or comment. The larger the amygdala the longer it will take to shrink it down.

The hippocampus

The hippocampus is primarily for memory — forming, consolidating, and reconstructing memories. It is heavily connected to our emotional alarm system (amygdala) and our perception part (thalamus), and their input affects how memories are formed. This is why two people in the same situation or at the same event can have completely different recollections.

Memories can change over time. They aren't static; they transform as we transform our perception. This is very important, because some people who have been a victim of a traumatic event, where the memory triggers anxiety and a stress response, think that they cannot change the memory associated with it, so they feel there is nothing that can be done. For people suffering from post-traumatic stress, the hippocampus replays back the memories in the form of flashbacks, but because the memory hasn't been effectively consolidated as being a past event, the person experiences the stress response as if the traumatic event is occurring in the here and now.

Learning how to bring the body and the heart into healing the brain and its memories is part of the way the brain and nervous system can re-tune into a calmer pattern. Memories can change and become consolidated in the past. We can learn to see a memory differently. We can transform a bad or traumatic memory into a post-trauma growth memory where we see the event as bad and we as the victim but can move into a space of acceptance and feel more agency within ourselves to respond differently if a similar event were to occur again in the future. Seeing the potential of trauma in this way can help us to understand that we can learn to process uncomfortable memories differently and that they can give us the opportunity to grow consciously. It is possible to move beyond them, heal the memories and develop new and more considered ways of dealing with it. The hippocampus is also involved in flexibility and using the things we know in new and innovative ways. When we are under chronic stress, the hippocampus shrinks, suggesting that our ability to manage memories effectively and be emotionally flexible and innovative reduces. Having a plump good-sized hippocampus is definitely something we should all be aiming for.

The thalamus

The thalamus is like the central station for the sensory input coming from the body, through the vagus nerve. It starts the processing of this information and then sends it out to the rest of the brain for further facilitation and interpretation.

Because the thalamus is closely connected to the hippocampus and the amygdala, our emotions and memories play a role in the input of the sensory information, and therefore impact our perception. This is so important to understand: perception is the experience of life itself. People who suffer stress therefore have a 'negative' stress filter that impacts the perception of a particular interaction. This is why a person who is generally kind could be perceived as threatening or untrustworthy by another. The cues of their altruism are not being picked up. Vice versa, those who have experienced chronic stress may not be as alert to someone who is not trustworthy. Their ability to pick up on that person's dishonesty and suspect behaviour would be less refined.

In Part 3, we move further into the solutions for settling down stress, anxiety, and burnout. By doing more body awareness exercises, which strengthen the communication within the limbic system, we can become more in tune with and trusting of the perceptions and sensory input systems of the body. Trust and safety are the foundations of anxiety, burnout and stress management. Firstly, we must trust ourselves and find safety in ourselves, only then can we find safety in others.

NEURAL REAL ESTATE

The brain lives very snuggly inside our rigid skulls. It reshapes according to experience, but it doesn't get bigger in some areas without shrinking in others. So the more stress we have, the bigger the amygdala gets — often taking some of the neural real-estate off the hippocampus.

Just like you can't make more earth, you can't make more brain, only change its use.

"What you pay attention to grows" is a remarkable truth in any area of learning, personal growth and brain and body awareness. As you start to de-stimulate the body or help the body to re-tune itself into a calmer state, you are in effect teaching the body that it is possible to attend to itself. [10]

When you are in a state of stress, or simply failing to attend to the body's need for rest or relaxation, you naturally go into a state of defence. By re-shifting the attention and understanding and accepting the body's need for rest, calm, peace and joy, we learn to regulate the brain and the body. If you want to develop the skills to recognise your own physiology and become a co-contributor to your health, you need to learn the necessary skills to realign your nervous system.

Exercise: Tending And Befriending

Take a moment to tap into your body, right now. Check your breath. Check your posture. Check your mind. Check your heart.

Take a long, slow, deep breath out. Make the exhalation longer than the inhalation. Do this five times.

Tune into the rationale of making time to learn to self-regulate yourself. Just like in sport or in business, if you want to get better at something, you must practise. You need to embrace this.

Simply sit back and ask yourself: "How can I find some time simply to attend to my body's needs?" Tension, a racing mind and irritability are simply signs that the body is defending itself against a real or (most often) imagined stress.

Tune in and listen to your breath. Imagine a shy child that is waiting for a sense of comfort before they find the courage to speak up and tell you what is wrong. Be gentle on yourself, and if you can't muster gentleness, just imagine yourself being kind. Most of us rush through life, tuning in starts now. Take some time to simply let the breath breathe itself. Checking in, just as you would with a sick friend. What is it you need from yourself? Let yourself listen. It could be you need more or less sleep, a holiday or simply to lie down and read a book. You might need to commit, make more effort, call yourself out on something.

The answer or the message may not come instantly. This is very common. See if you can stay simply with the sense of tending and befriending yourself, giving yourself the time and permission to honour you, all the good bits and the not-so-good bits. This may be the first time you have ever thought this way about yourself. Be kind, just as you would to that shy little kid who is trying to pluck up the courage to ask for what they need. Give them the space they need, no rush.

Ask yourself for permission to find the time to relearn your physiology and retrain your brain. Learning to regulate the body is the same as learning a new software program. I know you have the basics already. But if you want a body that is free from stresses and anxiety, a body that feels safety and in harmony with its environment, then these plug-ins are the equivalent to the premium package — this is the gold standard we all ultimately desire. Anything less is unworthy of the pursuit of aliveness.

Homeostasis is the overriding principle that allows the pres-
ervation and regulation of the flexible stability required for
optimal functioning of the body's physiology. This is a constant
fine-tuning of the balance of chemicals, temperature, pressure,
energy and hormones to make sure every part is doing its bit
to survive.

Homeostasis takes a lot of energy, especially when the body
is under stress. Therefore, we can be in a state of cellular
inflammation and not know it, as the body is trying to adjust
the internal environment to the external all the time.

The more we can offer an efficient and low-stress internal
world for ourselves, the better the body will work and the
longer we will likely live. Pretty simple and inspirational stuff!

Key Points:

- ✐ **The amygdala is known as the alarm centre of the brain and grows in response to chronic stress.**

- ✐ **The hippocampus is the area which stores memories; the more active the amygdala the less active the memories get laid down.**

- ✐ **The thalamus is the place where we collect all the information from the body and filter it through our emotional centres and memories to help us perceive the external and internal scenarios.**

- ✐ **How you perceive a situation is critical to how you respond.**

- ✐ **Automation of habits is a key evolutionary skill of the brain.**

- ✐ **Automation helps the brain be efficient with its energy requirements.**

- Automation has a negative side, as we are at risk of automating our emotional reactions, which can limit our personal evolution and negatively impact relationships.

- What you pay attention to becomes the foundation of your lived experience.

- Befriending our emotions, even the uncomfortable ones, can help us find a sense of internal safety and paves the way towards self-understanding and retraining the brain towards balance and optimal functioning.

chapter 15

THE AUTONOMIC NERVOUS SYSTEM

"We cannot solve our problems with the same thinking we used when we created them."

– Albert Einstein

I know I already have pushed my luck on the fancy scientific words of all the various parts of the brain, but this section is seriously important for you to understand, as the autonomic nervous system is a far-reaching system. It is either in protection mode (sympathetic nervous system) or relaxation mode (para-sympathetic nervous system).

The protection mode is an instant response to a threatening situation either real or imagined. The relaxation mode doesn't automatically switch on, it needs to be under intentional control. This makes sense because we don't want the relaxation system kicking in automatically when we are 100 metres from safety. Remember the baby monkeys and the tiger.

Let's dive in.

THE SYMPATHETIC NERVOUS SYSTEM

The sympathetic nervous system (SNS) is driven by adrenaline and is stimulating and activating. It is primarily involved in the fight and flight response. When this system is activated, either by a threat in our environment or an internal trigger like an emotional memory, we take up the position of being primed to protect ourselves.

Our nerves, via neuro-chemicals, stimulate the muscles to fire up. Our pupils dilate, our heart rate speeds up, our breath gets shallow and quicker, blood gets diverted to our brains and away from our kidneys, reproductive organs and digestive system (we don't need to be getting horny nor hungry at this particular time!) The immune system gets primed for inflammation and readies to repair an injury that might occur. Sugar gets pumped into the blood stream as an easy energy source.

A few moments after this cascade floods the body, the adrenals release cortisol. This is known as our stress hormone, but really it is all about trying to protect us from the impact of stress on the body. Every morning the body gets woken with a pulse of cortisol, getting us ready for the day. It gradually decreases throughout the day and stays low overnight. Cortisol stays high in response to chronic stress, to try to bring back balance to the body.

The risks of living in the jungle without permanent shelter and with wild hungry animals roaming the hills are not common these days. Most of us have set our lives up to have less random threatening events, but of course they still happen — natural disasters, terrorism and family violence are examples. However, most of the stress we feel is driven by our internal response to the threat that we are perceiving. This is different for everyone. For example, one person can live quite comfortably on $70,000 per year, and another will feel like that is poverty. Past experiences, resilience and expectations all play a role in how we perceive the stress we are facing, real or imagined.

By understanding the function of the SNS and how the flood of adrenaline and cortisol impacts the body, the symptoms associated with chronic stress can be understood as well. Stress not only lives in our minds, but it lives inside our bodies too. You may experience physical symptoms such as chronic muscle tension, temporomandibular joint strain, tension headaches, functional hypoglycaemia (sugar cravings, drops in energy, fatigue), chronic inflammation and pain, high blood pressure, asthma, irritable bowel syndrome, unexplained fertility issues, lowered immunity, recurrent infections, irritable bladder, insomnia, and hyperactive thinking, to name a few. By understanding how this works, we start to be able to become the witness to our own stress response and begin to feel empowered about choosing to do something about it.

The big difference between real threat and chronic stress is the response we take. Either fighting or fleeing is part of the natural way of discharging the chemicals inside our bodies. Some of you will know how effective a run or a work-out is in helping you feel more relaxed. We release cortisol and adrenaline during the work-out and increase endorphins (which are morphine-like chemicals) which help to create a more pleasant feeling in our bodies.

The neuro-biology of trauma[11] reveals that those who have the capacity to run away from the threat fare better than those who are not able to retreat, feel trapped, or watch on in frozen shock. Running away, such as the thousands of people running across the Manhattan Bridge toward safety on the morning of 9/11 terrorist attacks, or fighting for your life is the natural activation system of the body. Activating the biological self-protection system generates a feeling of agency and control inside the body which helps the person to makes sense of the situation, giving them an opportunity to protect themselves from further danger and preventing them from further psychological harm. When a person is a victim of significant trauma such as a natural disaster or an act of war, rape or other forms of abuse, the more damaging response is that of freezing. When the body feels overwhelmed and the person is unable to find the agency to self-protect — ie they are made powerless by their abuser, or pinned under a fallen structure — they have a higher risk of PTSD as compared to those who were able to find some form of protection for themselves and seek safety.[12]

The sympathetic nervous system command centre is essentially the amygdala. When we are under stress, burnout or anxiety for prolonged periods, the amygdala gets bigger. This means inside us, we have a bigger and louder and more sensitive alarm system. When this occurs, the alarm goes off at the slightest trigger — a snigger, a remark, an extra piece of work, a loud noise, a telephone ringing, a tone in another person's voice. We become hypervigilant.

Under chronic stress and anxiety our SNS is primed all the time, flooding us with chemicals. We feel constantly wired, on edge and irritated. This state of imbalance can therefore be associated with fatigue, lowered mood, low libido, easy weight gain, sugar cravings, poor concentration, low self-esteem, low confidence and poor sleep. Sound familiar?

Cortisol is intimately associated with the sugar and fat balancing hormone insulin. When cortisol is activated in times of stress, it sends a signal to the liver to make more glucose as an energy source. This then signals the pancreas to increase the production of insulin. Insulin then tries to regulate the glucose levels of the blood.

This is all well and good in acute stress where the body has time to repair and regulate itself after the distress is gone. However, in chronic stress the increased insulin stimulation can lead to increased production of fat tissues, especially around the abdomen. Therefore, chronic stress is associated with easy weight gain, fatty liver and increased risk of type 2 diabetes. Imbalances of sugar also leads to sugar and alcohol cravings, which then leads to further stress on the body. Here lies a little vicious circle, which needs to be addressed in the treatment of mental wellbeing.

The SNS is a beautiful system that has evolved over millennia to protect us from threat and help us to survive. It is important that we recognise that the stress response we are experiencing is in fact a protective and benevolent system that has our best interests at heart. By knowing this we can turn towards ourselves rather than away.

I can't tell you how many times I have heard people say with regards to their anxiety: "I just want to get rid of it." The sad part of that is you can't. You can't live without a stress response system. The more efficient way of dealing with it is to respect it, to take the time to consider what it is trying to tell you and take the time to start to listen to your body. Your body is your friend, and it knows what to do to heal you, but ultimately it is after teamwork. It wants the whole of you to lead the way.

THE PARA-SYMPATHETIC NERVOUS SYSTEM

Aaah, our relaxation response. The para-sympathetic nervous system (PNS) is almost like an internal massage therapist. It is a perfectly evolved system that is designed to calm the body and bring it back to balance. We can tune into it, and just like a muscle, it becomes more efficient the more we use it.

It is often referred to as the 'rest and digest' system. It is essentially operated by the vagus nerve, the longest nerve in the body. The vagus nerve starts in the brain stem (the reptilian area) and winds its way all the way from the facial muscles, tear ducts, eyes, salivary glands, and then onto the heart, lungs, liver, spleen, kidneys, bladder, immune system, pancreas, gut, and all the way down to the penis and scrotum in a man or the ovaries and cervix in a woman.

It is a bi-directional nerve, meaning it gathers information from all these organs and brings it back to the brain. It can send information to these organs and the face too. As the SNS activates in stress, the PNS plays the role of silencing a lot of these areas as required for the activation of the response.

In the West we rarely spend anytime considering the functions of the internal organs, they simply do what they do. By learning about the PNS, you will open an access point to the deepest parts of your body and develop a relationship with the body that is about fostering calmness, relaxation and balance.

The main access point to regulating the PNS is via the breath. The lungs are a vital organ and sit on both sides of the heart. When the breath is deep, full and rhythmic, it can regulate and modify the heart rate and blood pressure, sending a message to the rest of the body that it is safe to rest. Making your out-breath longer than your in-breath activates the PNS. This sends a message to the organs to relax, it stimulates the movements of the digestive system, it may stimulate the bladder to need to go to the toilet, and you may feel more sexual desire. Go you!

The PNS is connected to the anti-inflammatory aspect of the immune system, so when we strengthen the response of the PNS, we are stimulating our anti-inflammatory pathways. This is good news for those with chronic pain and for treating and preventing sub-acute chronic inflammation, a major underlying cause of heart disease, stroke, diabetes, depression and cognitive decline.

In an ideal world we would be operating in the PNS mode most of the time and utilising our SNS response only when needed. But this isn't the way our culture has set up our lives, so we need to consciously and proactively make time to activate the PNS daily. The good news is that we are all born for this.

Working towards improving the PNS response requires effort and time. Each time you consciously slow your breath down, tune into your body's needs, lengthen your exhalation or focus on gratitude you are strengthening your PNS, helping you become more stress resilient, flexible and calm. Most of the exercises you will learn throughout this book will activate the PNS. Unlike going to the gym, where we can quickly see physical changes to our muscles, neurons change and transform slowly. It takes a little more time and effort at the beginning.

Note that it is very important to feel safe from immediate harm, before trying to relax your survival mechanism. We will talk more about safety in Part 3.

OUR NEGATIVITY BIAS

We are primed to look for threat. If there were 10 different wild animals in front of us, we would scan them to look for the threatening one first, before we even bother to look at the benign ones. We remember negative things more often, we store negative memories more easily and retrieve them quicker. There is a common saying: we are like Velcro for unpleasant or dangerous memories and Teflon for joyful and pleasantries.

This is how we have evolved. It is more important to survive first and then thrive later. Thriving meant babies and the reproduction of the species — you can't do that with a dead or injured mother!

The trick here is not to deny this innate tendency towards storing negativity, but to work towards strengthening the opposite arm, the positive, so that we can assess our lives with more clarity, openness and sincerity. Negative experiences tend to make us feel contracted. We repel from negativity; you can witness your body pulling away. If we can teach ourselves to witness this and stay open to the negativity, we can see it for what it is, rather than feel dominated by it as we go about our lives.

This will help us navigate the changes we all experience in our lives. Life changes always, nothing stays the same. The great wisdom of the Buddha really stresses this point, and our lack of ability to cope with change often leads us to stress.

Exercise: Change Agent

Take a moment to think about your relationship to change.

Do you embrace it or struggle against it? Perhaps there was a recent event that triggered a feeling of stress in you. Could you change it? What would create the change in you? Was it because of the way a person responded to you? Do you have any influence over this?

Relationships can change, beliefs can change, our identity can change, our view of life changes, our bodies are constantly changing, our feelings can change, even our memories and perceptions of life can change. We have so much instability to deal with. Becoming adaptable to stress and being flexible is the key to honouring the changes we must endure all our lives.

Key Points:

- The autonomic nervous system has evolved to help us survive.

- The sympathetic nervous system (SNS) is activated when we feel threatened. It activates our 'fight or flight' response using chemicals and hormones.

- The para-sympathetic nervous system (PNS) is our 'rest and digest' system, that helps the body to return to balance after a stress.

- The main access point to the PNS is via the breath.

- Learning how to activate this part of the system allows you to gain more information from your bodily sensations and feelings to help guide healing and repair after trauma.

- As part of our survival evolution, we are wired to pick up threats more easily than positive feelings.

chapter 16

THE SOCIAL BRAIN

*"The self cannot be found in books,
you have to find yourself in yourself."*

– Sri Ramana Maharshi

We are wired for connection, and since we evolved from the higher mammals to humans, our skills in social integration and emotional development have significantly increased. In the pre-agricultural times, when many people across the globe led mainly hunter-gatherer life-styles, they used to travel in groups of around 150. This number is said to be optimal for social coherence. They worked together, bred together, grew families up together. Teamwork was a matter of survival.

The genes for social cohesiveness were passed down along the generations. Genes that promoted altruism, kindness, generosity and forgiveness have been shown to be essential features of human nature. For this to occur, brain and body pathways needed to be fostered and developed. In fact, social factors are amongst the most powerful influencers on brain plasticity.[13]

Empathy is essential to good relationships; the ability to imagine walking in another's shoes is vital. We all know what it feels like to be felt by another, and how good it feels to be understood. We do this understanding via our mirror neurons. These incredible little guys were discovered only a few decades ago, by Italian scientists Giacomo Rizzolatti and Vittorio Gallese. They are concentrated in the pre-frontal cortex and can be enhanced by meditation and personal development. They are like virtual reality stimulators of the brain and are involved in our empathic response to someone's intentions, pain or emotions. They help us see ourselves inside other people and see other people inside ourselves.

THE INSULA

There is another part of the brain called the insula, which connects the limbic system with the frontal lobe and other lobes of the brain. The insula is responsible for what we call introspection, an awareness of the inner workings of the body. Put simply, it helps us sense ourselves internally.

This connection helps us to read the emotions of others via our own filters. We can sense a person's emotions without knowing for sure or being told how they are feeling. The more we develop awareness of ourselves, our emotions, our sense of place and our emotional sensory system, the more we can detect it in others. Meditation has the potential to settle the neural noise that can allow us to sense, feel and see more clearly. For example, as we learn to recognise and settle our anxiety in ourselves, we can recognise it in others. This gives us the great gift of becoming sensitive to other people's emotions and paves the way for others to feel themselves too.

I have often said to some of my patients that my anxiety was my greatest teacher. It taught me to be sensitive to my own needs, but also empathic to the needs of others. It was a driver to fully engage in my life, and the lives of others. I hope by learning to embrace your stress, anxiety and burnout, you will eventually come to these conclusions as well.

Learning about these lesser-known parts of the brain will help you understand that by doing the exercises throughout this book, you can grow better connections inside your own brain. We know that practices such as mindfulness-based meditation can help develop feelings of care and generate compassion, and we know that even a short beginner meditation program can increase the density of brain tissue in the pre-frontal cortex.

THE PRE-FRONTAL CORTEX

I need you to know what is going on behind your third eye. This area of the brain is very important in who you think you are and how you behave. The pre-frontal cortex (PFC) is the part of the cerebral cortex that covers the front part of the frontal lobe. If you put your hand on your forehead, you will locate it perfectly.

This area is associated with our ability to plan complex things, to think our way out of a problem, to make complex decisions, and to manage our way around intricate social situations. It forms the bonds between our values, our goals and our thinking. For example, it helps us to differentiate among conflicting thoughts, determine what we think is good and bad, better and best, alike or different. It helps us assess future consequences with our present activities, work towards a clear goal, predict potential outcomes, and manage our expectations. We use this area to quash urges and modify potential anti-social behaviour.

It is somewhat easy to understand the functions of the pre-frontal cortex when we compare the teenage brain to that of a fully developed adult (some adults, anyway!) In the teenage brain, the pre-frontal cortex is still developing and won't be fully functional until they are 24-25 years of age. This means they rely more on their emotions than they do on rational thinking. When a teenager is really upset or emotional, it is harder to rationalise with them as compared to a more mature adult. This is part of why teenagers are prone to anxiety, impulsive behaviour, excessive guilt, emotionally-led decisions and challenges in planning ahead and reviewing all the consequences.

The pre-frontal cortex can quash emotional hyperreactivity and modulates the activities of the amygdala. Richard Davidson, a US-based neuro-psychiatrist, teamed up with the Dalai Lama to use MRI machines to study the brain differences between experienced meditators with thousands of hours of practise as compared to those who don't meditate or who are novices to the skill. They found a significant difference in the brains of meditators as opposed to non-meditators, showing that mindfulness meditation is associated with a thickening of the pre-frontal cortex, giving the meditators the ability to modulate the emotionality of the limbic system and to resist these to their psychological and social advantage.[14]

Key Points:

- We are wired for connection.

- Altruism, kindness and forgiveness are essential qualities in well functioning communities.

- The insula is the area between the limbic system and the pre-frontal cortex (PFC)

- The insula is like the mirror within us.

- The PFC can help us respond to a situation with more clarity, and awareness of the future impact of our choices and behaviour.

- Social behaviour is important in mirroring who we want to be.

chapter 17

CONNECTIONS BETWEEN THE HEAD AND THE HEART

"Only when head and heart work in harmony can we attain our true human potential."

– Jane Goodall

We as a culture conduct life through the lens of the rational mind, thinking and believing that intellect is far more important than emotional wisdom. We are a culture that reveres the ability to measure, prove and quantify. This bias disengages us from the more interesting, subtle and immeasurable part of our lives — choices, intuitions and knowings. Why we choose a path of creativity versus a structured, predictable roadmap of certainty, why we fall in love with someone unpredictably, why our choices are our choices, why we do the stuff that doesn't make sense to anyone else.

We know that both the head and the heart process information that impacts the body in a variety of ways, determines our responses to the events of our lives and maintains and supports our internal and external connections to the world and to ourselves.

The head tends to learn by pattern recognition. It takes past events in our lives and mixes them with current information coming from the body and the senses to create a way of approaching the world that makes sense to us. Pattern recognition is a vitally energy efficient process that helps us to cope with the dynamic nature of the world we live in. We are bombarded with so much marketing, media and information. The brain takes this and tries to make it as easy and streamlined as possible for us to cope with. Imagine if we didn't use our memories and patterns to support our lived experiences — every day as we got in the car, we would have to relearn how we drive and navigate traffic and steer clear of the people crossing the road.

But like all our incredible survival adaptations, pattern recognition can come at a cost if we utilise it without the whole in mind. For example, patterns can make us certain of things that are by their nature uncertain. Instead of seeing things from a new perspective, we make assumptions based on past experiences, locking us into the past, without us really knowing that this is what we are doing. This can form attitudes that can have long-term impact on our lives. "All teachers suck."

"I can't do math." "When you get close to people, they hurt you." "All men are only interested in one thing."

Let's face it, we do tend to pigeonhole not only ourselves but each other as we travel through life. This doesn't make us bad. It just means that we aren't fully giving ourselves the opportunity to assess new information, new relationships or new opportunities as effectively as we are capable. It is great to simply recognise that this is a fundamentally important part of our survival skills, but it isn't the only way we can choose to approach life. Giving ourselves the opportunity to renew or refresh our perspective can be helpful to our growth and transformation as individuals.

THE THINKING BRAIN

The brain loves patterns, stability, control and order. It helps us to manage our energy resources and, in a way, contributes to homeostasis. But sometimes when we want to transform our lives, find new solutions to old problems, or develop and change our attitudes and behaviour, the brain is not as forthcoming as other parts of our bodies. It can be a liability.

I have seen this so often in my work, especially the retreat work. When people start to develop a new sense of themselves or a new way of looking at the world, they can feel affirmed of a decision that will transform their lives, like leaving a job or a toxic relationship, only to be bullied back by the thinking brain.

I remember one woman, who had a PhD in biochemistry, who was so resistant to the subtlety of the more intuitive feeling sense. She commented: "I am just more scientific than that." Her intuitive sense was so unfamiliar and scary. She had relied so heavily on her intellect to survive and guide her through life that when she started to feel into a more holistic way, she would revert back to the intellect every time, despite her wanting to find a new way to approach life, minimise her emotional suffering and create meaning. Can you relate to this? Often when we can sense a flowing interconnection or an opportunity to lift off from the old into a new adventure, our head brings us back, into order, stability, practicality, structure, safety and old patterns.

Look around and see this in yourself and others.

A few years ago I read a book by Harold Kushner, a learned Rabbi, called *When All You Have Ever Wanted Isn't Enough*. It is a personal exploration of his choice to choose himself over the big, admired life he found himself engaged in. Outwardly successful, travelling the country, teaching thousands of people, but away from family and friends, away from the joy, the simple pleasures that make life rich and incomparable. After his son was murdered, this collision in brutality versus joy was the impetus for him to choose the quiet and soulful life, instead of the heady, brash and outwardly intellectual one.

As a physician and GP, I can admit that I have hidden behind my intellect, shutting things down, condemning them to the realm of lesser. I have put conviction, intellect, success and striving before my own joy and lived experience. It wasn't until I put my heart back in my life's broth of wonder that I truly could embrace both aspects of myself, letting the thinking mind do its thinking things, while also making space for the heart's subtle and strange songs. The combination is a profound mix of light and shade, yin and yang, poetry and words, art and science.

What I truly find wonderous is that we are born with all the neurons inside ourselves that we are ever going to get. It is simply the pattern of how they connect to each other that changes and develops over the ages and stages of our lives. We have this incredible ability to transform ourselves. Learning new things, thinking new ways, behaving differently, reviewing our old ways and choosing differently. This is not only for the smart ones, or the educated ones — this neuronal refashioning is available to all of us now.

This is why the sages say we can turn our lives around on a dime, in a millisecond. At any moment, we can choose a new way.

Exercise: Automatically Me

Remember the concept of automation? Just like physical things can get hardwired and become automatic, so too can our thoughts, emotional responses and behaviours. But if the brain is the pattern maker, who does the choosing? Where does this inner voice live? How do we develop a more independent and connected alternative to the pattern-making brain that rolls life out for us?

Is how I react, a representation of how I want to behave? Can I choose another way of being?

Over the next few days, carry these questions with you as you respond and react to daily life.

THE BAD NEWS, AND THE GOOD NEWS

"The measure of intelligence is the ability to change."

– Albert Einstein

Unlearning a skill, an emotional pattern or an unhelpful behaviour is not an easy thing to do. Can you imagine yourself unlearning how to drive? You might have a bit of understanding if you started a sport and taught yourself, only to find out your grip on the golf club for example is all wrong and that is why you splice every second ball onto the next hole and can't shift your handicap off 34.

Trying to change ingrained habits takes a lot of practise, but with determination and persistence it can be done.

Neurologically the heart and the brain are intrinsically linked. The heart sends messages to the brain via the PNS and the vagal nerve, to areas of the medulla (brain stem). This information then flows upwards into the limbic system and on to the pre-frontal cortex. The heart's messages can either inhibit the emotional response or activate it. The links to the more cognitive aspects of the brain show us that the heart's 'new and innovative' interpretations of the world can be fed into the brain's circuitry and modify previously held ideas.

The heart learns differently. It isn't direct, it isn't linear and it doesn't care for patterns. The heart is always scanning for new possibilities and new ways of being. It seeks new understandings and is intuitive. The head thinks, the heart understands.

Scientists and philosophers call this intelligence 'qualia'. Qualia is the experience of the feelings and qualities that is subjective to you; the quality of your experience as compared to another person's experience. It is still debated as to where qualia resides, but it is likely to contain aspects of both the heart and head's processing skills. Qualia is often associated with feelings of the more subtle kind, such as love, compassion, tenderness, forgiveness and gratitude. This is where the emotions have a definitive felt sense — you feel forgiveness, you don't think it.

When we are in these kinds of emotional states, there is an associated calmness, peacefulness and clarity, and the feeling can be felt throughout the body. It is like the mind opens into the space. There is a slowing down. This is naturally associated with feelings of hope, wonder, optimism and aliveness. The natural state of the body is peaceful.

The good news is that by practising attending and savouring these states of mind, states of the heart, we can strengthen the neural connections that support more ready accessibility.

Key Points:

- The head and the heart have bi-directional communication pathways.

- The head uses patterns to learn, react and automate.

- The heart uses symbols, senses and intuition.

- Attending to the ways of the heart requires patience, silence and listening to the subtleties.

- Qualia is the felt sense of the interaction between the head and the heart.

- Peace and calmness is the natural state of the human condition.

- The heart's interpretation of the situation can transform the brain's automatic response.

chapter 18

YOUR AMAZING BODY

"The constant flow of life again and again demands fresh adaptation. Adaptation is never achieved once and for all."

– Carl Jung

Maintaining integrity, balance and life is the key to the body surviving, reproducing and hopefully thriving. Thriving comes last. It is a little like Maslow's hierarchy of needs. We need to make sure we have the basics sorted to be able to grow into our potential.

The gut, brain and skin are an incredible triad of organs. Despite the skin being the largest organ of the body, the gut's surface area is eight times larger. If you were to lay out the gut end-to-end and open it up, the surface area would be about the size of half a tennis court.

The gut has been big news over the past decade and rightly so. It is a remarkable organ, which has the closest and most intimate relationship with the outside world. Its basic role is to break food down into micro-chemicals and nutrients, so that the body can absorb them. The fibre and other aspects of the food then get acted upon by the gut bacteria. The gut bacteria don't work alone and ideally work in a synergistic way. They coordinate the health of the body. They produce chemicals which we then absorb. Depending on what they are fed, they can be either good for us or not so good for us.

The gut ecology is vitally important for health, and how healthy it is depends on what food we put in our mouths. It is an extremely adapt-able ecosystem that can literally be transformed from good to bad and bad to good within 24 to 48 hours. A big night on the booze, followed by a high fat processed meal can be enough to set it off in the wrong direction for days, whereas a highly nutritious plant-based meal can be an elixir for the body.

Our culture is slightly devoid of revering the things we should revere. Where we admire busyness, success, and an expensive fast car, we should be worshipping organic heirloom vegetables, polyphenol rich food, kindness and extreme biodiversity in our food chain! I know it isn't very sexy or blingy, it probably wouldn't make anyone a vast wad of cash and it makes me sound like a complete geek, but understanding the vital nature of food and bringing reverence back to our soils, food production, cooking methods and the sacredness of sharing a meal is a vital component of health, community and sustainability.

BACTERIA

The gut isn't the only ecosystem of the body. We have bacteria everywhere — in our mouths, all over our skin, up our noses, in our vaginas and inside our ears. We are covered in bacteria that live synergistically with us. They are an essential part of our protection and our survival.

It is fascinating to think back to a time not that long ago when we didn't know that bacteria existed, and we certainly didn't know how intimate our relationship was with them. The pilgrims' arrival in America in search of a new land from Europe marked the first time in human history where a large bunch of young people left their families en masse. In the days of no contraception, many of these women got pregnant and delivered babies along the way.

Back in the homeland, midwifes had been part of the community, and were able to use their knowledge to assist the young mother to deliver. No longer having this option, the husbands, who had previously not been invited anywhere near childbirth, were suddenly thrust into a new role. Imagine not having seen or been around birth — the process of labour would be frightening.

Watching their wives in pain, the men wanted a way to see where the baby was at. For the first time in known history, vaginal examinations, un-gloved and with minimal running water, were performed. These examinations introduced external bacteria into the birth process. Women started getting infections and the maternal death rate rose. Without the knowledge of bacteria, nobody had any idea why these women were succumbing at such high rates. Decades later, in the mid-1800s, a young Hungarian obstetrician by the name of Ignas Semmelweis discovered the connection.

At that time, the biggest cause of death in women giving birth was infection. Early in the century it was at the rate of one death for every 100 births. After a policy change which stated that medical students and obstetricians also needed to perform autopsies as part of their duties, the death rate soared to nearly one in ten. In response, the Vienna Hospital opened another obstetrics ward, staffed with midwives only. The death rate returned to its previous level.

Semmelweis was curious, and on further investigation it became clear that the only difference between the two wards was that the medical students and obstetricians performed autopsies and the midwives did not.

At this time, the general thought was that diseases were transmitted by smells. It took another 20 years before germ theory was recognised. Semmelweis discovered the missing link, when his friend died of sepsis after receiving a scalpel wound whilst performing an autopsy on a woman who died of an obstetric infection. He joined the dots, realising that medical students and obstetricians were transmitting infections from cadavers to women in childbirth. A new contagiousness was established.

It is hard to imagine that hand-washing in between patients and procedures was not commonplace before this, nor were gloves commonly used until the late 19th century. It took another 50 years for the medical establishment to fully accept the role of hand washing and bacteria contamination as a source of disease.

THE IMMUNE SYSTEM

Shifting our relationship to bacteria can be life altering. The gut, the brain and the skin are derived from the same embryological tissue. This means they are inherently linked from the primordial cell layers.

In addition to the gut and the gut bacteria providing us with nutrition, it also provides the protective layer to block pathogenic bacteria, viruses and parasites from entering our bodies. If there is anything foreign that the body hasn't seen before, it will begin a frontline defence to protect us, rallying the immune cells and making antibodies against the foreign material. So important is this immune function for the gut, that two-thirds of our immune system originates in the gut layer. These immune collections, called Peyer's patches, line the small intestine.

The immune system protects us from the outside world, as well as from the inside world. It helps to balance our inflammatory pathways and achieve the delicate balance between inflammation and anti-inflammation. It is closely connected to the brain in relation to this. The immune cells have the same receptors on their cell surface as the brain cells. They can cross the blood-brain barrier and go wherever the brain directs them to go, but they also bring information back to the brain to further the inflammation or to send the signal that it can be stopped.

Our immune system and our digestive system are responsive to the same chemicals inside the brain, such as melatonin, dopamine and serotonin. In fact, there is more serotonin in the gut than there is in the brain, which is why anti-depressants that work on this area can cause gut dysfunction. It is also why sub-acute low-grade inflammation is associated with depression.

When we are stressed, anxious or experiencing burnout, symptoms such as irritable bowel, brain fog and skin eruptions are common. Eczema is commonly exacerbated by stress and strongly associated with gut inflammation and gut ecological imbalance. See the interconnections?

THE STRESS RESPONSE

When the body is stressed, it requires more energy and nutrition to remain in balance and to perform ongoing tasks. Just like during the

COVID-19 pandemic crisis, when we needed more hospital beds, more staff and more oxygen. When we are stressed, however, we are also losing more nutrients. Nutrients such as B vitamins, vitamin C, magnesium and zinc all get used up more readily in times of stress as compared with states of calmness.

Often when we are stressed, we turn to things that can give us short-term gains, but ultimately lead to increased stress. Take caffeine for example. Often if we are stressed, we are using up our brain sugars more and we aren't sleeping that well at night. We are fatigued. We rely upon caffeine to reset our energy. It is a stimulant, like adrenaline, and therefore activates our sympathetic nervous system. Caffeine increases magnesium excretion via the kidneys and we lose magnesium with every cup of coffee we consume. In addition, we are too tired to exercise, so our intracellular mitochondria aren't as fit, and we feel fatigued with exercise rather than better. We are too tired to cook a meal, relying on takeaways or processed foods or sugary easy-to-get meals (which are devoid of nutrients such as magnesium, vitamin C, zinc and B vitamins). We are wired at night, so we take to drinking a few glasses of wine, which depletes our magnesium and B vitamins. So we consume fewer nutrients, consume more things like caffeine and alcohol, which further deplete our nutrients — and we use more nutrients in the process of trying to maintain balance. This further exacerbates our feelings of strain and stress and makes us feel even worse than we could. Stress and our response is the ultimate vicious cycle!

The gut is served by what we consume, but how it functions is also determined by our thinking mind and how much stress we are under. It responds to internal stress the same way it responds to external stress. When the stress response is activated, its functioning is altered and the immune system goes into defence mode.

Stress hormones such as adrenaline speed up the peristalsis temporarily, often causing diarrhoea. I'm sure some of you would be aware of this connection, but under chronic stress, the dysfunction in the system and the drawing away of blood flow from the gut can create constipation. This 'on again, off again' stress response is in part why some people with irritable bowel syndrome get diarrhoea, some get constipation and some get a combination of both.

When we are under an acute stress, the gut can cease functioning, to aid us in shunting the blood to more vital organs to defend ourselves. This means the gut shuts down temporarily. Under stress we often don't feel hungry, or can feel easily full. This dysfunction can impact on the messages sent to the lower bowel. The upper gut (stomach), when filling up with food, sends a message via the nerves of the gut to the lower bowel and gut bacteria to get ready, and this can often stimulate a bowel movement. Under stress this messaging system doesn't work as accurately.

FOOD FROM NATURE

The reason we attribute such power to the gut is multi-layered but somewhat misleading. The power of the gut depends upon the food we feed it. The food provides information for the body, but it also feeds the gut bacteria which make substances that can enhance health or decrease health. The foods we choose to eat impact the quality of the information that the body receives from the outside world. Eat junk food, get junk messaging. Eat food that is nutritionally charged, get optimised information. When we get good information, the body can operate in a better way, allowing the messages to be clearer. This can help the brain function better and we get more clarity.

More clarity (which is a function of the pre-frontal cortex) allows better connection to the nervous system and the heart. The more clarity we have, the more we see, assess and attend to life with accurate responses, rather than reactive automation. This in turn equates to better immunity, better mood, better sleep and better choices. How easy is that?

When the body is fed well, the nutrients provide the basis of the chemistry we are beholden to. The body feels safer and more in control of its reactions and responses to life. So, in part, what we eat aids our autonomy, and our relationship to the whole. This is not about being perfect, as we are all imperfectly perfect, it is about nourishment and acknowledging our intimate relationship to nature. Food that comes from nature allows that nature to come inside us and helps to protect the cycle we are a part of. Fake food, processed in factories, devoid of nutrients and energy, depletes our bodies and nutrients, and negatively impacts the information sequencing required for optimal health.

If we fully embrace the concept of food being information for the body, then we can choose along those lines and gain yet another way of supporting ourselves to optimise our mental and physical wellbeing.

Key Points:

- The gut, skin and brain are intrinsically linked and all act as the barrier between the inside and the outside world.

- The immune system shares the same chemical receptors as the brain cells. They have a bi-directional communication network.

- Melatonin, dopamine, serotonin and adrenaline all impact the immune system.

- Acknowledging the role stress plays in disrupting homeostasis and its impact on the functioning of the gut, the immune system and the brain is essential for effective treatment.

- Food provides information to your body and brain. Better food choices = better information.

- By increasing support to the gut (via dietary choices), the brain can help support homeostasis via sleep, relaxation and decreasing mental and emotional stressors.

chapter 19

GUT FEELINGS AND INTUITION

"The intuitive mind is a sacred gift and the rational mind is a faithful servant. We have created a society that honours the servant and has forgotten the gift."

– Albert Einstein

Think about the last time you had a gut feeling. It is often referred to as an intuitive feeling, a sense of something that is intangible and often difficult to explain in words. Did it make you feel good, or wary? Did you respond to it or ignore it?

A gut feeling is a feeling inside your body, felt mainly in the abdominal region and generated by the autonomic nervous system. It is a top-down message that is beyond the rational thinking brain. It might involve things like tummy rumbles, feeling tight in the stomach, or butterflies in the tummy. It can also lead to feeling squeamish, vague discomfort, nausea or retraction, constriction, a pulling away.

A gut feeling isn't always indicating danger. It can indicate a positive leaning into a situation. It is a misnomer to call it 'gut' feeling, because it is the information coming from all the organs innervated by the vagal nerve. It is perhaps more accurately called body wisdom, or the heart's intuition.

Whatever you call it, this innate sense provides visceral information that is beyond our thinking mind. Because of this, it doesn't always concur with what our rational mind thinks.

The more we are tuned into the body, the more we can learn to trust it. When we are practised in only using rationality in our lived experience, we can be very materially and linearly successful, but not necessarily in tune with our heart's desires. This can lead to a pervasive feeling of discontent.

By bringing in the whole of the body and accepting that the viscera (the organs) have a role in communicating to the inside and outside world, we can respect and honour all the emotional expressions, information and nuances available to us to live our lives.

A body with optimal communication, that is in harmony with the external environment and internal environment, is a body that operates at ease and with flow. This is akin to living in tune with yourself, nature and your ecology. The internal fighting settles down and the natural joy and contentment has room to rise. This is what the Buddha calls our first nature, our innate nature, which is founded in compassion, joy and kindness.

In our culture, we tend to live out our lives in isolation, us against the universe, a dog-eat-dog kind of worldview. One that is devoid of a sense of connection to nature, let alone a sense of connection to the universe. But as a scientifically obsessed culture, we seem to miss the fact that we can't not be connected. Tuning into this connection with not only ourselves but to life and to land and nature in general is the only pathway to the aliveness we all crave.

Dr Mary Graham is a Kombu-merri woman and Associate Professor at the University of Queensland's School of Political Science and International Studies. She is a world-renowned expert in Indigenous and non-Indigenous forms of knowledge and Aboriginal history, and talks of the need to develop a relationship with the land ahead of our relationships between people. This counterview to Western culture is contingent on the Aboriginal belief of the importance of land to life, the sacredness of the land and the fact we are born from the land and will return to the land upon death. She has said that "for Aboriginal people, land is the great teacher; it not only teaches us how to relate to it, but to each other; it suggests a notion of caring for something out-side ourselves, something that is in and out of nature and that will exist for all time".[15] She talks about the law of obligation, coming into a sense of integrity with our responsibility to look after our foundations, one of which is nature itself.

We all have an opportunity to tune into ourselves and the planet. If we honour this relationship, it can support us when times are tough for us or for those we love. To look towards our body's innate wisdom, which is synergistic to the innate wisdom of the land. Next time you are walking in your local forest or watching the sunset, tune into your body or to the world around you and ask for support, for interpreta-tion, for acknowledgement that inside of us, inside our connections, is a wisdom that is beyond our intellect. It houses the guidance we all so often search for.

If we trust this 'gut feeling', it becomes a viable way to regain and re-trust our autonomy, mystery and unique role we all play in life.

Exercise: Riding The Waves

Take a moment to settle in. Make your body comfortable. If you are close to a park or a green space, immerse yourself in it. Firstly, tap into your breathing. Allow your body to settle. You might like to place your hand on your heart or your belly or both. As you start to settle, just coach yourself into saying that it is okay to tune into your body right now.

If there is discomfort with this, simply acknowledge the discomfort and take this as information for yourself. Allow yourself to unravel. Let your shoulders rest, let your buttock muscles relax and allow your jaw to slightly fall open.

As you tap in, tune into all your abdominal and pelvic organs. Take your breath down into the pelvis if you feel comfortable. You might like to send a little greeting to your stomach, your bowels, pancreas, liver and kidneys, your womb, your prostate, your genitals. Even if you have a poor relationship to any of these organs, see if you can come to a sense of peace, an amnesty of sorts.

Now open your eyes very quietly and look around, with a sense of reverence and just simply look into the landscape. If you are in an urban setting, you can simulate this by playing some nature sounds and looking at an image of a rainforest or similar.

Try to see this landscape as if for the first time. Look around with reverence. If you start to feel uncomfortable and bothered, again acknowledge this resistance and see if you can stay a little longer. Try to take in the details, the grass, the insects, the breeze, the trees.

See if you can sense what the Aboriginals feel in relationship to the land. See if you can go a bit further and bring the nature within you. See if you can ponder at the intelligence of life, the way it goes about itself. By tuning into nature, we are tuning into ourselves. It is the symbiotic relationship that guides us into our knowing.

Now come back to your body sense, your organs. See how they are feeling, talk to them, notice any resistance you have towards any part of your internal milieu. Breathe and send yourself some warmth and encouragement.

You are one, you belong. You are the custodian.

Key Points:

- Gut feelings are also known as body wisdom.

- Looking after our true nature is key to acknowledging what is greater than us and what sustains our health.

- Gut feelings, when trusted, can help guide us through life.

part 3

LIVING THE WONDER WITHIN

chapter 20

ACCESSING YOUR INNATE HEALING SYSTEMS

"What is aliveness?
It's hope. It's possibility. It's freedom."

– Esther Perel

This section is filled with guided exercises and concepts to help you navigate the wonder within. Because we are working on the whole body, all the exercises interrelate. They assist each other in strengthening the skills required to develop a more heart-centred approach to living and relating.

There may be some exercises you connect with right away, some you feel less comfortable with and others which you feel have no impact. Watch your reactions, resistances and comfort levels with curiosity and an open mind. If you feel agitated, annoyed or frustrated, see if you can stay present and be gentle with yourself. Know that these emotions are entirely common and expected at times.

Sometimes you will have to do the exercises multiple times to activate the subtly we are trying to achieve. You may do an exercise easily one day and feel like you reach a new level of peacefulness only to wake the following morning feeling uptight, annoyed and bothered. You may progress well for a few days and then feel like you have a setback. This is quite normal too and we will explore this in more detail a little later in the chapter on pitfalls.

Know that it is in the repetition that the real magic is activated. Just like learning any new language, it is going to take time to listen and to attune yourself into yourself.

It is the wonder within, and there is no direct route. It is like you have been given a recipe book written in a foreign language. Your job is to tune in and create the recipes that will give your life zest and spice and help you lay out a feast for all the world to see.

FIND SAFETY FIRST

Please do not attempt any of these exercises unless you feel safe in your body. This is particularly important as safety is a primal experience;

without it we can't truly relax into retraining our neurological system and body into a new way of relating to the world and ourselves.

Find a place where you feel safe, at home, in nature, by the ocean or anywhere that suits. It is like a refuge — it could be your bed, in a bath, by your favourite tree, reading a book, with your pet or walking on the beach. Make sure you are comfortable, warm and won't be disturbed.

If you feel better when a person or animal is around, keep them close. Starting with mindfully patting an animal can be a great way to deactivate an over-active nervous system. The more you can pay attention to the settling of your nervous system, the more you have conscious control over it. See if you can regulate your breath when you are patting your beloved furry friend. They will love it too.

If you don't have an animal, you can either borrow one, use a soft toy or a pillow, or even use an imaginary one. Feel or imagine how the animal touches you back. Focus on its real or imagined movements: your cat purring next to you, your dog snuggling its head into your body, your horse pushing its head into your hand.

It doesn't matter how long it takes you to find some safety, please make sure you really focus on this. If you are not an animal kind of person, you can do this exercise with a pillow, or even just gently finding safety inside yourself using your own touch.

Safety is the key to doing this work, but for some it is harder to find than for others. Anxiety often feels like a perpetual state of feeling under threat. If this is an issue for you, I suggest that you work with a trauma informed counsellor, psychologist, doctor or yoga practitioner. You may need to go very slowly. Pace yourself, you are engaging in a new way with yourself. Start where you are and continually tune in with yourself to make sure you are okay.

If you are very anxious, try going for a walk outside before doing the exercises. A walk can help you become centred and feel more present. Each time you modify yourself towards calmness, it gets easier.

LABELLING

Labelling is a foundation exercise that can be done anywhere and anytime. The next time you feel a strong emotion, try this exercise out.

E-motion = energy in motion. When you have an emotional reaction, be it pleasant or unpleasant, it floods the body with chemicals. The whole body experience can feel overwhelming and all-consuming.

Exercise: Labelling What Is

Simply labelling the emotions you feel, as you feel them, can have a profound effect. You can do this by saying it in your head, out loud or even writing it down. Try things out for yourself and see what works for you.

Once you find the label that feels right, such as "I'm feeling fearful", "I'm feeling overwhelmed" or "I'm feeling really angry", keep repeating it. Try to stay present with how you feel in your body and acknowledge the emotion as a simple matter of fact.

Remind yourself that even though these feelings are very uncomfortable, it won't cause you harm to feel them.

Labelling engages the whole brain in the emotional response and brings in the awareness of the frontal lobe. This can activate the forward-thinking capabilities we all have and can broaden our response if we find the emotional reaction is neither helpful nor appropriate.

Emotions are felt in wave forms, that pulse throughout the body via the messaging of the heart. Even though we experience the emotion as if it will last forever in the immediate phase, it will in fact dissipate in its intensity. As time passes the emotion will naturally fall away.

As you become more adept at witnessing this, you will come to see that this is the very nature of our emotionality as a species.

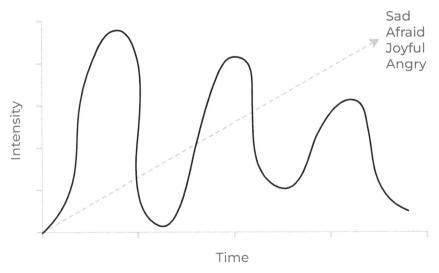

Holding and witnessing fear - its natural rhythm.

The straight line indicates what we think will happen when the emotions are intense. The curved line is the natural energetic wave pattern of how emotions flow.

THE CONTAINER

I want to introduce you to the concept of 'the container'. Think of your body as a container, which you need to look after first, before you look after anyone else's. You know this rule from travelling on a plane: always fit your own mask first before you attend to your child.

We only have authority and control over ourselves. We can't control nature, each other, our children, our partners, our staff, our boss, our parents, our colleagues or our friends. We can at best try to influence them, but we are not responsible for their lives, their habits, their patterns or their behaviour. You are responsible for your life, your habits, your behaviour and your choices. And you have the power to make changes to these responses. This is the most empowering information you will ever receive.

Exercise: What Is It Going to Take?

As you contemplate the journey inwards, ask yourself: if not now, when?

Take a moment to ponder this. What is it going to take for you to change what is no longer serving you?

As you linger on these thoughts, perhaps more will come. You may come up with practical issues, emotional resistances or fears about judgement from others. You may not feel skilled, equipped or empowered.

See if you can take this opportunity to ask yourself some further questions: is this true? What else do I require?

No one can do this work for you. You have more pathways to wellness than you realise. They are not always obvious, promoted or supported by those around you, they can challenge your sense of being 'cool' or 'tough', but they aren't expensive, they are always available, they perfectly match your innate biology and once you start repeating them, they can become a framework for a better relationship with life, yourself and all the people you choose to have in your life.

You must start where you are. In the words of Rumi, "if all you can do is crawl, start crawling."

You are nowhere else but here, and you have got what you have got. Working on your container is something you can start to do right now. There is nothing else you need to start the journey towards wholeness.

So, if you are ready to begin, read on…

chapter 21

THE BREATH

"With every breath I plant seeds of devotion.
I am a farmer of the heart."

– Rumi

I cannot tell you how underrated the breath is for healing. Despite this being so well known, it is hardly ever emphasised as one of the most important and critical factors in your health. The breath is where the gold lives. Through practise it will become the most accessible way for you to assess, recognise and analyse how you are in every situation that you choose to tap into.

As Rumi alludes to in the poetry above, the breath is the way to the heart. It is the field that the heart grows into. It provides the oxygen that is like the sunshine to the seed. I have spoken to many people about the importance of the breath, but it is only those who truly embrace it, or even dare to come into a friendship with it, who begin to create a landscape that will help them nurture the growth they seek.

The lungs provide the cradle to the heart, the heart nestles inside their rhythmic arms. They are the yin to each other's yang and are in a constant relationship with each other. When we fall in love, or see something of beauty, our visceral reaction — felt through the heart — can literally take our breath away.

In a world where we rush through our days, often arriving slightly breathless, we go from task to task in little conscious communication with our internal sunshine. We breathe shallowly and quickly. A little like the African missionaries we rush so fast over our lives. The breath helps give us an opportunity to reclaim our space.

We breathe about 18,000 times per day. Every breath offers us the chance to choose another way. The breath is always in the present moment, never in the past or the future.

You can activate the para-sympathetic nervous system — the rest and digest aspect of your body — by consistently focusing on increasing the length of the out-breath and making this longer than the in-breath. This sends a signal to the body that it is safe to relax and the calming process can begin.

Exercise: My Gentle Friend

Take a moment to do this now. Breathe in and out five times. With each breath you take in, slow the out-breath down. How do you feel?

When you first start to attend to the breath, you may become a little anxious. Sometimes if we are not used to tuning in, when we start to watch or observe ourselves, it can feel a bit strange, and for some people it feels overwhelming. Sensing yourself slowing down can feel unfamiliar. Your breath may be tight, erratic, not rhythmic as you would like it to be. Can you take the pressure off it to be a certain way? Can you just watch it? Try to simply see it for how it is. Don't try to change it. Welcome your breath as an old friend.

See if you can lengthen both the in-breath and the out-breath now. Lengthening as well as deepening is key. See if your breath feels only in the chest, or if you can bring it into your abdomen as well. As you breathe in, see if you can push the breath into the pelvis, all the way down to the genitals. By opening the breath into these areas, you naturally create a vacuum that allows you to deepen the breath.

One of the key factors I have learnt about the breath is that it is innately very gentle. It is innately kind and it seems to settle just by us giving it some attention.

Stress and anxiety tend to make us breathe shallow breaths, and if we are triggered often, we hold our breath a lot. Watch yourself over the next few days to see if you stop breathing when you feel anxious, in a panic, or overwhelmed. Tune in with the aid of your breath to see how your jaw feels.

Look a little at your breath. Do you lose your breath with very little exertion? Even when talking? Do you feel that you freeze or hold your breath? Does your chest feel tired and fatigued even though you haven't exercised hard?

In these exercises the trick is to observe first, then become aware, before you start modifying. This is very important. Many people jump to 'trying to get it right'. There is no right or wrong in this process, it is simply you observing yourself as the curator of your body, becoming aware and then modifying as you need to. If you simply jump in and modify based on another person's advice you risk giving up too soon or losing the awareness that is central to more long-term change.

It is just like what they teach you in a first aid course. First assess the situation for danger or risk. Then respond. We as a culture tend to jump in, no assessment, loosely follow the instructions without any reverence of their validity, and then if we feel no effect within a few minutes, write it off as a load of crap. I know you know what I mean or know of people who do this all the time. We need to stop doing this as we are now in an epidemic of stress, anxiety and burnout. All is not well in our world; as individuals and as a collective we need to start grabbing this stuff like our lives depend on it, because they actually do.

TAPPING INTO YOUR BREATH

Cardiorespiratory synchronisation (another term for heart-lung connection) modulates and influences the brain, activates the parasympathetic nervous system (PNS) and dampens the response of the sympathetic nervous system (SNS).

Stress, anxiety and depression are associated with increased dysfunctional breathing patterns. As you know, the stress response is meant to be a short-term defensive approach to aid our survival when under threat. When the acute threat dissipates, we ideally return to a state of calm and rest and bring ourselves back into a harmonious state of homeostasis.

Mindfulness meditation, diaphragmatic breathing exercises and yoga influence this cardio-respiratory synchronicity, which affects the energetic oscillations of our brains. The breath alters the energetics inside our cell membranes, and this change then affects all the cells within the body and brain, influencing the return to a homeostatic state.

Another way to assess the effect of the breath on the whole body is by assessing a person's heart rate variability (HRV). This is a measurement of the beat-to-beat changes of the heart's rhythm. A high HRV measure is suggestive of better health of the PNS. The HRV is a measure of the balance and adaptability of the autonomic nervous system (the SNS and the PNS). When our autonomic nervous system is in sync this can lead to more regulation of the upper cortex of the brain and the whole body. When the HRV is both high and smooth, the body goes into a state of coherence. Coherence is a state where the cells are at maximum efficiency and productivity. As we practise exercises such as the ones in this book, we can achieve higher HRV and coherence and therefore better health. When a person is using a deep, slow, abdominal breathing pattern, this is positively associated with an increase in HRV.

Exercise: Yoga Breath

These are four ancient yoga breathing exercises that help in de-stimulating the SNS and activating the PNS. Try to do one of these per day for the next four days and see what effect they have for you. Do you feel one is more effective than the other for you? You can also use these as a recovery tool in the event of an acute stressor or to help you sleep at night or to settle your mind down before bed.

1. Abdominal/diaphragmatic breathing

Abdominal breathing is generally done lying on your back. Start with one or both of your hands on your abdomen. To take an abdominal breath, inhale slowly and deeply, drawing air in so your hand rises. This might take a bit of practise if you are normally a shallow breather. Your belly should expand and rise as you inhale, then contract and lower as you exhale.

If you are having difficulty, you can do this lying on your tummy so you don't have to breathe against gravity. Try to stay with this exercise for five minutes.

2. Alternate nostril breathing

This is very effective, especially to help still the mind and for sleep issues.

Hold your right hand near your face. Start by placing your right thumb over your right nostril. Breathe in through the left. When it is time to exhale, open the right nostril and close off the left nostril with your right index finger. After exhaling, inhale through the right nostril and close off the left with the thumb again.

Repeat this process for five minutes.

3. Breathe-in, breathe-out a hum

A hum is a low steady buzzing sound like a bee. Humming on the out-breath has an incredible stilling effect, by exacerbating the vibrations within our bodies. Close off the lips and make a humming sound as you breathe out.

Tune into the vibrating feeling inside your head and throughout your body.

Set yourself a timer of 5 to 10 minutes.

4. Box breathing 4:4:4:4 or 4:7:8

Box breathing is a way of focusing the breath in a rhythmic fashion. There are two options to try.

Breathe in for four counts, hold for four, out for four, hold for four. And repeat for 10 cycles of breath.

Or, breathe in for four, hold for seven and breathe out for eight. And repeat for 10 cycles of breath.

If I haven't already convinced you of the superpower of your own breath, I want to set you a challenge. Every time you start a new task, take a breath. Every time you put the key in the door, go from one situation to the next, take a breath. Before you eat, take a breath, before you answer the phone, take a breath. As you listen to another person, or a song, take a breath. Every time you login to your computer, take a breath. When you stop at the traffic lights, take a breath. If you are like a stranger to your breath, just start with getting to know it a little more, start to become the witness to your own energy source.

Ask yourself:

- How do I feel when I lengthen my out-breath?
- Can I do this without anyone knowing?

Your breath is your secret weapon. It is your vital connection to the present moment that can open your senses and provide a doorway into the synchronisation with your heart.

Key Points:

- Cardiorespiratory synchronisation modulates the brain, activates the para-sympathetic nervous system and deactivates the sympathetic nervous system.

- Heart rate variability is a measure of the adaptability and balance of the autonomic nervous system.

- Befriending the breath is vital in the management of stress, anxiety and burnout.

chapter 22

TOUCH

"Touch brings presence home."

– John O'Donohue

The breath is the essence, but what we can achieve via our skin, our spatial awareness and our social touch system is equally as remarkable.

Did you watch the Netflix documentary called *My Octopus Teacher*? An incredible story about the wonder and intelligence of the octopus. It begins with a depressed, burnt out executive who retreats to the sea to find healing. During his daily cold-water plunges, he seemingly befriends an octopus and develops a relationship with this intriguing creature that uses skin receptors to feel its way around, and uses touch to connect. I watched on in wonder.

We have these skills too. We all have this inbuilt capacity to feel the world around us. We are as wonderous as the octopus.

When I was in medical school, I went to extensive lectures exploring the microscopic world that lies just below the surface of our skin. The skin is the largest organ in the body, providing a protective barrier to the outside world, keeping us inside, in a nice package we all call 'us'. Our skin is filled with receptors that engage constantly with the outside world.

I remember learning about the nerve cells that sit underneath the skin, bringing in information about pressure, pain, temperature and light touch. Is it hot or cold? Painful or pressurised?

There are also an incredible number of neurons that are dedicated to interpretating our spatial awareness; how we know where we are in space. This ability to recognise spatial awareness is also called proprioception. Proprioception provides us with a sense of ourselves in this world, even without sight. Try it now. Get a cup of water and put it in front of you. Now close your eyes. Wait 10 seconds. Can you locate the cup of water? This is proprioception at play.

Proprioception is literally our sixth sense. We don't ever turn this off — even when we are sleeping, we are subconsciously aware of where our body is. When we lose touch and proprioception, we literally lose the ability to control the body.

When we are stressed, anxious or in burnout, we do not lose proprioception, but we rarely focus on it either. Our awareness is often on the stressor, the threat, or our own anxieties and fear. The brain is firing in the state of self-protection, and we can even become more clumsy, stubbing our toes, bumping into walls, hitting the side of the car on the kerb. This reduced awareness is common in people suffering from stress.

Proprioceptive receptors are located in joints, muscles, tendons, ligaments and skin. They constantly feed an incredible amount of sensory information back to the brain. The sensory input area of the brain is very large to accommodate this constant information gathering.

BODY AWARENESS

Like a musical instrument, body awareness is the activity that literally tunes us into the world. This is a way to heighten our skills on observing, locating and becoming aware of the subtlety that lives inside our skin. The body scan exercise outlined below is one of the starting points for all mindfulness practise.

I must admit when I first started learning mindfulness and was recommended to do this exercise for 10 minutes every day, I found it incredibly boring. But knowing that it is impacting a huge part of my brain and modifying the information that sits between the frontal lobe and the limbic system, I started to get a little more interested, a little more curious and a little more motivated to get on and make sure I was doing it regularly.

Over time my relationship to body awareness training has transformed. I really look forward to tuning into my body and finding out which bits feel particularly tense. I feel a great comfort in my ability to let the stress go. I start every meditation session with a sense of focus on my body, where I am in space and how it feels. Body awareness went from boring to interesting to downright empowering. It didn't happen overnight mind you, but with practise, gentleness and a bit of commitment, I feel confident in maintaining the quality of my relationship with my container.

Exercise: The Body Scan

Sit in a chair, with your back straight and your feet touching the ground. Use one of the breathing exercises above to allow your body and mind to settle. Say to yourself: "There is nowhere else I need to go and nothing else I need to do right now." Repeat this if you are feeling restless or resistant. You could play some music to help create some space or light a candle or some incense.

Start by focusing on your feet. Feel your feet on the ground, focus on any sensations in your feet. If you feel you need more grounding, tap your feet on the ground a few times and notice what that feels like. Feel the temperature in your feet, the difference between the soles, the tops and the toes. Feel the sensation of the connection of your feet on the ground.

Now move your attention up the legs, to the calf muscles. Feel what they feel like, notice them in the space, tap into the sensations. Can you feel the tingling? Can you imagine the blood flowing?

Then let the attention come upwards to the thighs, home to the largest muscles and bones in the body. Feel the strength of your thighs as you give them some attention. See if you can feel their warmth, their sturdiness. Tap your thighs to feel them, flex and relax the muscles.

Now come up to the pelvis and start to bring the attention to the pelvic bones, the muscles that hold the hips together, the buttocks and the internal organs, such as the genitals. Feel whatever you can feel. What happens if you relax the muscles a little more? Feel the sensations of the chair, as it supports you. What does your back feel like, coming up from the stability of the pelvis? Focus on the internal organs. Can you bring some gentle attention to this area and send it some gratitude for all that it does for your body?

Now bring your attention up the back, feel the back straight against the chair. Rest back a little bit. Rock forward and back — can you find more comfort for yourself? Imagine an imaginary string coming from the top of your head connecting you to the sky. This helps to lengthen the spine, which is a more energetic pose for the body to sustain.

Now bring your awareness into the shoulders. You might like to move them around and feel if you can relax them more. Can you feel the sensations of the shoulders, or any vibrations or temperature changes? Can you feel how your clothes feel against your skin?

Now bring your attention down your arms. Feel the arms as they hang from the shoulders and come into focus on your hands. Feel your hands rest on your lap. Feel the temperature changes; perhaps your fingers are cold or warm. Take some time to bring respect to your hands. They help you so much. They help you touch and love the world around you.

Come up to your head and your face. Can you relax the muscles around your eyes and face? Drop open your jaw. Is it tight or tense? Try to relax your tongue. See if you can relax your face totally. Let all the tension drop away. Can you relax even more?

Now bring your awareness to the front of your body. Start with the torso. Feel your belly, as it breathes. Imagine all internal organs all working silently inside you. Can you relax your tummy muscles?

Now bring your awareness into your heart space and lungs. Really focus on the breath and the way the ribs and chest rise and fall. See if you can feel your heart beating for you. Visualise a soft light or essence coming from your heart. If you can't visualise it, imagine that it is there. See if you can feel the gentleness of your breath. Explore your breath. See if you can spread that essence around the whole of your body.

Now come into the whole of your body. See your body sitting in the chair, take in all the sensations you are feeling: the chair, the floor, the breath. Any tension you feel, see if you can let it go. Feel the whole body breathing, beating, vibrating.

You might also like to try this exercise, which uses labelling to allow us to tap into what is.

Exercise: I Am

Sit up straight in a chair. Start by tapping into your breath and coaching yourself by saying: "There is nowhere else I need to go and nothing else I need to do."

Start with stating the facts.

I am sitting in this chair. I am feeling the chair and how it is sup-porting me. I am feeling my feet on the ground. I am relaxing my muscles. I am breathing more deeply. I am letting go of tension. I am sensing my body. I am attending to my needs. I am learning how to relax. I am looking after myself. I am taking my mask off. I am letting tension in my face go. I am being grateful for my hands.

Take it from here. What else can you add to the sentence "I am..."?

Do this for five minutes, to help train the brain to be aware of the present moment.

By tapping into my body's awareness system, I was able to strengthen my sensory ability to tune into how I felt and how I was reacting in time and space. It forms the border between my felt sense and my aware-ness, my sensory cortex and my frontal lobe and my lived experience.

The other role of proprioception is to quickly find our body in space, so we can respond more quickly with an action/motor plan. Tuning in with more sensitive attention to the body awareness fortifies our ability to respond with more autonomy in our lives.

THE SOCIAL TOUCH SYSTEM

Touch is a very complicated sense, and we use it more than any other. We are constantly subconsciously scanning and touching our bodies for lumps, bumps and wounds. Touch is the way we feel life occurring to us; our skin contributes to our very experience of our life. We say things like "they feel good" or "he is a cold person", or "she has a warm heart". We metaphorically bring the enormity of how we tacitly sense the world.

Did you know that if I snuck up behind you and moved a single hair, you would immediately know it? The sensitivity of this system is awesome. In many ways, the sensory information we get from our bodies and skin is more wide-ranging than the information we get from our eyes, ears and mouths.

For instance, heat and cold sensation work on different nerves than light touch sensations. Pain, itch and pressure are distinctive also. There are some touch sensations that are completely dependent on the context that you feel them in. Think of the touch you feel from a tickle from a lover compared to that of a stranger. Same feeling, different experience.

This is called the social touch system and it is vitally important in our learning of love, safety and connection. Tapping into the social touch system ourselves can be a great starting point to accessing a sense of safety and connection with ourselves. Even though we touch ourselves all the time, bringing conscious awareness of this touch can be transformational in the relationship we have with ourselves.

Neuroscientists are coming to understand that touch and proprioception are vital ingredients in consciousness itself. They are vital in forming our subjective sense. This is the aspect of mind that creates our unique interpretation of the world. It is like mind and consciousness is a sensory soup of awareness, mixing our sensory inputs — like touch, smell and proprioception — and combining them with our emotions, thoughts, memories and our predictions about the world. This soup is what generates our consciousness. A whole sense of self emerges from these separated systems, that create a form greater than the sum of its parts.

Mindfulness supports this process. We start to practise getting back the sensation needed to find our own sense of support. When we lose our awareness of our body, we lose the container needed to help guide us through our lives. Therefore, body awareness practices are the cornerstone of the mindfulness process.

Here are a couple of great ways to tune into touch.

Exercise: Loving Touch

Start by simply placing one or both hands on your heart. Take a moment to focus on the touch you feel in your hands and the touch you feel on the skin of your chest. Tap into the sentiment you are feeling right now. Can you, via this touch, enhance a sentiment of care for yourself, of trust, or of simply connecting?

Now bring your hand to your belly. What does this feel like? Can you feel your breath? Can you feel your gut?

Now bring your hands to the opposite arms. Try stroking your hands down your arms, softly, like a loving massage or tickle. You could squeeze some light pressure across your shoulder with both hands, to give yourself a little hug. What does this feel like? If it feels foolish, remember, this is just for you. No one else is watching, and no one else is allowed an opinion. We are in an epidemic; we have no time to waste holding ourselves back from ourselves!

Does giving yourself a light touch or holding your heart feel good, helpful, calming or relaxing? What else might you feel?

Key Points:

- The skin has direct access to the brain and the heart.

- Body awareness exercises increase the pathways between the limbic system and the pre-frontal cortex.

- Self-activating the social touch system can increase a sense of safety and care in our bodies.

- Social touch and proprioception are key ingredients in increasing consciousness.

chapter 23

THE HEART'S DOORWAY

"Your heart knows the way,
run in that direction."

– Rumi

Entrainment is a process through which independent systems interact with each other and come into harmony with each other. The body does this by using the oscillations of the heartbeat to synchronise all the different parts and different systems together. In addition to the heart-beat, oscillations are found throughout nature and determine things like cell-to-cell communication, flowering in plants, circadian rhythms and ovulation cycles.

When our systems work together in a harmonious way it dramatically increases the body's efficiencies. It brings greater clarity, enhanced intuition and people report simply feeling better. In a state of harmonious entrainment, we can also start to gain a sense of being at one with things outside ourselves, like nature, other people and the universe. When the heart rhythm is in a state of coherence and the heart is feeling enraptured in senses such as appreciation, love and gratitude, the heart in effect entrains the brain. In these states, we come into a state of being in sync with ourselves. It is in this state that healing is said to occur.

Attaining and sustaining states such as this requires practise to the point that it becomes familiar. This isn't always easy, as the brain loves familiarity. It loves the feeling of knowing what to do, when to do it and what is going to happen next. It is this top biological survival adaptation of automation that makes it hard for us to change old, ingrained patterns; sometimes the brain fights like an old dog to keep what has been safe and sound for it for a long time, even if these patterns cause problems in our lives.

The trick is to try to get the head to surrender to the heart long enough for it to be able to decipher the mysterious and often elusive messages that it brings. The heart's wisdom is cryptic and wordless. The heart is beating and fully formed before any brain cell is made. It is through the neurons of the brain that speech occurs. The heart doesn't use words to communicate, it uses senses and feelings and whole body awareness. Therefore, it is the combination of starting to become in tune with our breath, our skin and our senses that we can start to decode and understand the heart's guidance.

You might have heard the saying that "the brain thinks and the heart knows". The brain uses analysis to manage life, the heart feels authentic and deep. The brain is where our intellect is, and the heart is where our intuition and sensitivity live. The heart feels light, expansive and joyful. The brain feels safe, reliable and practical. The brain loves concepts. The heart loves truth. The mind is the incredible relationship in between.

We all know of times when our head has overruled the heart in relationships, career decisions, friendships and adventures. But maybe there have also been times when all logical and rational thinking told us to do the safe thing, the one that involved less risk, the tried and true path, but there was something inside that guided us to take a chance, make a bold move, turn towards the unknown and jump.

When I was 27, I was somewhat stuck in a relationship that had gone stale. His life was going in one direction and I was yearning for another. We would talk about adventure and moving across the other side of the world for a while, but nothing was shifting. One day I called a friend who was in the travel industry and booked a ticket to Paris. When I arrived in Paris a week later, my life was thrust into a completely different paradigm — just think *Eat, Pray, Love*. My time in Paris (and also Spain) was one the most transformational periods of my life. I travelled with my heart wide open and my mind witnessed an expansion that was poetic and wild. New ways of thinking, new opportunities — like seeing the Dalai Lama present his first speech to the Western world in Barcelona in 1999.

Nine weeks later I arrived home, and my brain had convinced me to stay in the old relationship. It was safe, familiar and he was reliable. I convinced myself that staying was the right thing to do. I had had my fun and it was time to settle down. But life had other plans for me. A few weeks later, I found myself alone in my apartment. My boyfriend had left me. Then the phone rang. It was an old friend, Will, who I hadn't spoken to for months. When he heard about my break-up he offered to come over, and half an hour later I heard his crazy old car's muffler roaring up the street. He bounded up the front stairs, swept me into his arms and said, "I'm taking you out for dinner!" At 1:00am as he dropped me home, my brain was no longer trying to rationalise the irrational. Nine months later I moved in with Will as friends. Six weeks after that, we started dating and 21 years later, we are still happily married.

In hindsight, I now know that the rumblings, restlessness and frustrations I felt before booking that flight to Paris were messages from my heart. The feeling of stuck-ness, of needing to get out, was a symptom of my heart feeling congested and imprisoned. I had tried many things to deal with these symptoms: trying to reframe my relationship, look at the positives, get myself fit, focusing on my female friendships. But the deep longing remained inside. It was, in hindsight, undeniable, even though I was trying very hard to deny it.

I couldn't see the future, I couldn't see Will waiting in the wings, so the pull towards the new was frightening. But the combination of being pushed and being pulled is often characteristic of the heart's execution.

Key Points:

- Entrainment is the process of independent systems coming into harmony with each other.
- Synchronisation is determined by oscillations.
- The heart is the key oscillator of the human body.
- When we are in sync, we are more efficient and optimised.

chapter 24

TAPPING INTO THE HEART

"The moment you accept the trouble you have been given, the door will open."

– Rumi

The heart loves truth. It loves silence and stillness. It is inherently shy and easily over-ridden with the slightest pretension, busyness and brazenness. It is patient, it is kind, it is mysterious and it can be bolshy. It can be hard to read and at times it feels like it doesn't make any sense. Its essence is gentle, still, authentic and sincere.

The heart has a delicateness to it, but this is not akin to being fragile — far from it. The heart is a workhorse. We must fight against the illusion that the delicate ways of the heart are soft or weak, and therefore insignificant. To do this would place us as a victim of the cultural imbalance that rejects these qualities in many arenas of society.

The HeartMath Institute has done many studies using HRV as a guide to ascertain which states help bring about coherence and entrainment within the body. Find the space and courage to tune into yourself and see for yourself the effects these manifested states can have on your psyche and your body. When you discover what works for you, you will begin a profound and personal journey into a meaningful new relationship. There are three states we will explore: appreciation, self-compassion and love.

APPRECIATION

Even when we are in a state of stress, anxiety or burnout, or just feeling overwhelmed or out of balance, there is usually something we can focus on that we appreciate. It can be as simple as a hot cup of tea, a warm blanket, a refreshing swim, a beautiful tree, a colourful sunset, a message from a loved one or the wagging tail of a pet. Simple things like this feature in all our lives, and even when we are feeling resentful, angry or hurt, we can still tune into something of grace that we can appreciate.

Let's do this now.

Exercise: Warming The Heart

Choose one thing to focus in on.

I like to choose a member of my family. I remember one of my girls as a little child, and think back to when they went and picked flowers in the garden for me. Other times I place myself in my mind on a big rock that I have sat on, looking out to sea or on a mountain top. (Don't worry if you can't muster anything. I have been in your shoes before. If you can't find anything to be appreciative for, just imagine that you feel appreciative.)

Sit back and focus in on that sense of appreciation. Place one or both hands on your heart space and see if you can attach the image in your mind's eye and bring it into the heart, just like the heart is feeling it. Allow your breath to settle. Feel the breath rise and fall.

See if you can imagine the sense of appreciation getting bigger with each breath, and filling and warming the heart. See if you can share this sense from your heart space and make it feel like it is being delivered around the body via the blood flow. Like you are sending appreciation into your tummy, down your legs to your feet, up your back, across your shoulders to your hands, up into your face and then returning to the heart. Flood your body with appreciation.

See if you can muster a slight smile and savour this feeling.

Take as long as you like with this exercise. When you finish, take a moment to tune in with yourself. Was it challenging? Did you sense a resistance? Was your mind busy? Do you feel better? Do you feel slightly more relaxed? Did it feel nice? Was focusing on a nice warm shower easier than a relationship or vice versa?

Whenever we start doing these kinds of exercises, it is important that we start to learn how to sit with whatever comes up for us. In my experience, often the feelings that I resist offer the biggest lessons in hindsight.

I recently attended a retreat, as a participant. I listened as a woman in my group spoke about a 'life dream' she was working on. She would move to a small island and live a simpler life, riding her bike around town and hosting long dinner parties with beautiful food and wine. I was fond of this woman, so I was very surprised to realise I was feeling annoyed by her 'syrupy and frivolous' dreaming. I sat with what I was feeling. It was clear I felt envious and resentful. As the day went on, I continued to feel really bothered. Why was I feeling so envious? Why was I feeling so annoyed? I went to bed that evening with the same feelings, wondering what the emotions meant for me.

I woke the next morning with strong feelings, what I felt as a kind of grief. The retreat facilitators set a task: we were to meet up in small groups of three and talk about the day before. We had 10 minutes to speak freely, and our partners just had to listen. At the end they could give feedback on what you said. As I started to debrief, I brought up my feelings about the woman's story. As I was talking it out, I came to a realisation. I felt annoyed that she could grab onto life and feel its joy, but I was holding back from it because I feared finding my joy. It felt like joy was okay for others, but not for me; as a doctor I had a responsibility. I realised I feared truly jumping into my life.

My two buddies stood there listening, silently. I could tell on their faces they were shocked by what I was saying. To them I was so vibrant, so alive, so present, and here I was telling them I was scared to fully embrace my freedom. Shani, my partner, grabbed me, by the shoulders, her eyes wide. She bellowed in the finest Indian accent: "Live, Michelle, fucking live!" As she spoke, I could feel fear rising. I knew then that it was the thing that sat underneath the annoyance and the envy. It was a profound roundabout way to gain more access to deeper fears. Staying with the body, the emotions and just being curious to their intensity provided an incredible opportunity to encounter my own truth.

Shani's words have become a mantra for me; a reminder that my fear of freedom, despite my yearning, is real. It needs care, attention and love. Stepping into ourselves is not clear-cut, easy or quick. It is not without confusion or illusion. It is not linear, and it runs on a time period that is completely at odds with any scheduling we have. So, you need to stay with yourself, and stay true to what you are feeling. If you feel angry, feel angry. I don't mean go out and yell at someone or punch a wall, but see if you can watch and inquire as to why the anger has come. Has a boundary been overstepped? Has someone disrespected something you believe in? Are you in relationship with someone whose values oppose yours? Has the anger triggered a fear of abandonment? Is your anger in fact sadness or a response to loss?

The process of coming into your heart allows you to develop courage and be attentive to these incredible things we call emotions.

SELF-COMPASSION

"This kind of compulsive concern with 'I, me and mine' isn't the same as loving ourselves. Loving ourselves points us to capacities of resilience, compassion and understanding within that are simply part of being alive."

– Sharon Salzberg

Respecting the need for self-compassion is one of the most important parts of this inner work. Many of the incredible teachings of this work can be lost because of this almost paralysing disregard for the needs of our deeper selves. This is ironic as we live in such a self-obsessed world, where narcissism is on the rise. But self-obsession is vastly different to self-compassion. Self-obsession is a divisive state, one that says "I'm better than you", whereas self-compassion is inherently inclusive — "we are all important, including myself."

We are all innately compassionate. It is our baseline. When we all go through a crisis together such as a natural disaster like the bushfires or a COVID-19 lockdown, people rally together. We mostly activate into being of service to those less fortunate than ourselves. In lockdown people got slower, kinder and more responsive to each other. Neighbours were checking on neighbours, dropping meals around to those suffering or unable to work. We naturally think of other people, and it feels good to be able to help.

It is often argued that some people are not innately compassionate — the greedy corporates, the thieves, the narcissists — but this is not their true nature. Their apparent lack of compassion for others is usually nothing more than a case of a hardened heart. It is a response to trauma or fear of not belonging. It is beyond the scope of this book to discuss the ramifications of trauma in depth but closing off from others and going into defence mode is often a way of protecting ourselves (rightly or wrongly) from life, love and connection.

Just as compassion is innate to being human, so is the experience of suffering. Suffering is as natural to life as breathing. We all suffer. It can be as common as being left out of a shared group chat, or being dumped, betrayed or disbelieved. Sometimes we don't get the job, we fail an exam, we let other people down, we make a bad decision, we fall out of love, we do a dumb thing and get caught, we mistreat someone. We all do it. I do it, you do it, your friends and loved ones do it, enemies and strangers do it. We all make mistakes, we all betray each other and we all suffer consequently. We can often acknowledge mistakes in other people, but in this culture of 'stiff upper lip' we tend to ignore our own suffering and just carry on. We either ignore our pain, disregard it or belittle it as worthless. The standards we impose upon ourselves perpetuate our suffering, and on and on it goes — until we find another way.

Many people see self-compassion as self-pity, even confusing it for self-indulgence. But self-compassion does not mean my problems are worse than anyone else's. It is simply an acknowledgement that I am human too; I have needs that are equally as deserving as others and my lived experience is as valid as another's. Self-compassion creates an equal playing field.

To learn how self-compassionate you are, visit www.selfcompassion. org. This is the website of sociologist researcher Dr Kristin Neff, and it contains a validated questionnaire you can complete in around five minutes.

Self-compassion is a tool that can foster a deep sense of belonging to the self. By embracing and accepting ourselves we can fundamentally be more available and present for others. Starting with the self is the most selfless, sustainable and effective tool we have. If our leaders, health care practitioners, business owners and politicians could embrace the concept and the practise of self-compassion, we could transform the landscape of the world.

Self-compassion has been scientifically validated to improve our emotional wellbeing and contentment. It fosters a positive mindset, and is associated with less destructive patterns of fear, negativity and division. When we are anxious, stressed or burnt out, our decisions are often made from a place of fear and contraction. Self-compassion allows us to open to our suffering and expand into the discomfort, rather than shrinking in the face of it, running away or hiding from it. Self-compassion is a pathway to fully becoming human. Self-compassion is an invitation to be who you are and to open your heart and mind to the world. Self-compassion allows us to start where we are at. We start with practising kindness to ourselves. You are, right here and now, good enough.

Exercise: Write Yourself A Letter

Find a quiet space where you won't be interrupted. Imagine yourself as a little child, in a place that is familiar, perhaps your family home, kindergarten or primary school.

Imagine yourself feeling anxious or upset. Perhaps you are in trouble, have done something wrong, or somebody has hurt you. Write a letter to yourself like you are your own best friend, a kind caregiver or even an imaginary loved one.

Reflect on how this little child is feeling and write out what you would like to say to them. How will you guide them into the future, what wisdom will you share? Perhaps you can focus on some strengths that you see in them. Think about the context they find themselves in and share with them your understanding, and your desire for them to be happy and healthy.

After you have finished the letter, take some time to reflect. How does it feel to offer care, and how does it feel to receive it? Try to let the words sink in. Notice if you are resistant to the words of kindness. If you are struggling, offer yourself some kindness. If you don't drink it in now, when are you going to start?

I am what society would call a success. I won the lottery with a good education and a good brain that suited the current educational system. I am happily married and I live in a safe land, with good health care and opportunities. I had good self-esteem. I got a medical degree, and I ran a business that was successful.

But I was a hard taskmaster, with no self-compassion. It wasn't okay to make a mistake, it wasn't okay to fail, it wasn't okay to slack off, it wasn't okay to say no to those who needed my services and it definitely wasn't okay to ask others for help. If other people wanted to blame me for something, I took on that responsibility — I should have been kinder, more generous, more thoughtful. If someone complained about me, I took that on too — I should have known more, I shouldn't have asked so many questions, I shouldn't have cared. I even gave myself a hard time for caring too much.

Bringing myself into the equation, and allowing myself to become kinder, softer, gentler and more understanding to myself, was one of the most fundamental shifts I have made on this little journey I call my life. Please, I implore you, share your generosity, kindness, care and empathy with yourself. Not because you are better than anyone else, but because you are alive and you are the only one who can do this for yourself. You can love, respect and honour yourself, just because you are human.

Self-compassion is actively offering ourselves self-care. In a world without self-compassion no one wins.

Exercise: Let The Love In

This exercise is a seriously humbling, seriously effective and seriously gorgeous way to explore the wonder within and journey towards better self-compassion and optimising your relationship to your core. Please don't tell anyone else about this exercise. Nobody needs to know about it. In fact, it is important that they don't because you don't need anyone else's approval to love yourself. Developing a relationship with yourself is a very intimate affair, and just like we don't share the intimate details of our love affairs with others, it is best to keep these moments sacred, shared only with you.

Look at yourself in the mirror, with or without placing your hands gently on your cheeks, like you would as a loving gesture to a small child. Lean in closely and whisper to yourself that you love yourself. See if you can repeat it once or twice. See if you can hold your gaze. Don't put any pressure on yourself, just try it and see.

Now wrap your arms around your shoulders, like you are giving yourself a hug. Squeeze tightly and focus on how this feels for yourself. Stay with yourself.

Do this every day for a week, even twice a day or more if you get the inclination. Each time you do it, I want you to tune into how you feel and simply keep doing it.

When I first did this exercise, I felt very shy and embarrassed. Offering myself some kindness and some affection felt completely at odds to my previous relationship with myself. But as the week went on and I continued, my embarrassment turned into giggles. I started to feel like I was having this love affair that was hidden, exciting and forbidden. Further into the week I noticed I was feeling more comfortable with the experience. I felt I no longer needed a mirror and could simply place my hand on my heart and send myself loving, kind thoughts. I was blown away with how incredibly quickly I could transform a feeling of failure or humiliation into a loving experience of humility.

SELF-LOVE

Self-love is not pampering. It isn't going for a massage once a week or getting a facial (although there is nothing wrong with that). It has nothing to do with indulging the pleasure senses. Self-love is respecting your boundaries, putting your own needs on the table, making sure you have enough for yourself as well as others, and protecting yourself from those who impose on you in an overbearing or disrespectful way.

This fierce form of self-love is often a challenge for people to understand and activate, because it appears to be at odds with the limited image of love that we absorb through our literature and film. That love is soft, sweet, kind and gentle. Yes, love is all those things, but it can also have a ferocious, fiery and intense side to it. It is like love has both a yin and a yang aspect to it. When you think of the yang of love, think of the fierce love of a parent who will do anything to protect their child. It is love fuelled by a loyal fire. There is no permission needed to activate this kind of love. It is fearless, unapologetic, untamed.

The yin-yang of self-compassion

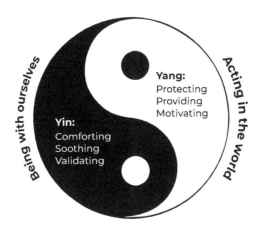

Image credit: Neff, K. D. & Germer, C. K (2018).
The Mindful Self-Compassion Workbook. New York: Guilford Press.

Jefferey Pfeffer, a Professor of Organisational Behaviour and author of the book *Power*, writes that "belief that the world is a just place anaesthetises people to the need to be proactive in building a power base". He encourages every person to make sure they seek power as if their life depended on it. He uses terms such as 'personal agency' and implores us all to make sure we stand on our own two feet and fight for our right to be here, to be present and to achieve a sense of personal empowerment that is neither defensive nor apathetic, but merely a true expression of our worth, our agency and our influence. Some of us feel uncomfortable about claiming our space as if it is arrogant. Self-love requires a personal determination for oneself, that we may need to fight for ourselves, fight against the power of the inner critic and stand up for ourselves like we never have before.

Exercise: Love Me Tender, Love Me True

Take a few moments to contemplate what kind of loving style you like to portray.

Can you imagine loving in a different way? Does your inner critic pipe in and judge you for how you express your love? Does your love ever appear as intense or fiery? Do you repel this kind of emotional response?

Asking yourself these questions can allow you to open to a more complete understanding of love and most importantly how to love yourself.

Caveat: It is common to confuse obsession with love in intimate partner violence. Violence is never an acceptable expression of love. For more information regarding violence and abuse in an intimate relationship call 1-800-RESPECT.

Some people love through their actions, others their words and others their intentions. Some people love fiercely and others love gently. Our expressions of love can look completely differently depending on the circumstances.

Self-love is both fierce and gentle, wild and kind, fearless and humble.

Perhaps by allowing ourselves to be ourselves (a fine act of love) we can allow more acceptance, more permission to express what we feel, and slowly release ourselves from judging our emotions.

Exercise: Meditation Of Self-love

Make yourself comfortable, either sitting in a chair or lying flat on your back. Place one or both hands on your heart. Play some music that is calming and creates a space of comfort for you.

Take a few minutes to let the breath settle, coming into the observation of the breath. Feel your whole body in space and take a
few minutes to scan the body. Where you feel tension and stress,
encourage your muscles and body to let it go. Don't forget to scan
your face. Let yourself come into a comfortable position.

When you have done that, come into focusing onto your heart space.
Take a moment to settle in here and see if you can tune into the energetic essence of your heart. As you take in your longer and slower
breaths, imagine the heart enjoying the gentle cradling massage from
the lungs.

When you feel ready, see if you can either visualise or imagine a
light surrounding the heart space, like it is bathed in sunlight. The
colour of the light can be any shade you like. If you have trouble
imagining, just tap into the desire to imagine it. Let this light grow in
intensity with each breath you take. When your heart is bathed in
this beautiful light, imagine this light starting to ever so gently and
ever so slowly travel down inside your heart space, spiralling into
the deepest parts of the caverns of your heart. As it spirals down, just
watch and witness the gentle glow of your heart.

Breathe.

In a few moments you will arrive alongside the light to the centre
of your heart. Allow the light to open into the most beautiful and
calm space.

Breathe.

Take a look around. Sense the stillness and the wisdom within the
heart space. Allow this sense to fill the body.

Breathe.

In the distance, you see a person, standing inside the cavern. As you
notice them, they turn around and you see that the person in front of
you is you. If you feel safe, walk a little closer so you are face-to-face.

Please take some time to look into each other's eyes. In this moment of connection offer yourself a greeting, a hello, a welcome, a gentle acknowledgement. Reflect on what it feels like to be facing yourself, inside your heart space. Whatever it feels like, just let it be. There may be resistance, or even a shyness, hurt, sadness, relief. Whatever is there, is here. Stay with yourself.

If it feels okay to do this, ask yourself a question. You may also like to offer yourself a promise, like "I'll try to connect with you as often as I can", or even make a statement, like, "Thanks for sticking with me". Whatever feels right for you in that moment.

Breathe.

Linger for a little longer now, as you sense a quality from the question, promise or statement. Perhaps a word or a sense may come forth between you two. Whatever arises, see if you can make space for the connection. Ask yourself: how does it feel to make this connection?

Linger a little longer and let the sentiment, feeling or promise soak throughout the body. Let it start to flow beyond the walls of the heart space and see if you can feel it flowing down your legs or up into your face and hands. Acknowledge how that feels and take another breath.

As you prepare to come out of the meditation, acknowledge the relaxation you have created in your body. Come back into feeling yourself in the chair or lying down on a bed or floor. Bring a small amount of movement to your feet and hands and as you do this, really tune into the slight movements you are making.

When you feel ready, open your eyes and take some time in slowly moving the whole body before you sit up.

Key Points:

- Self-compassion is key to acknowledging the power of your aliveness, your strengths, weaknesses, vulnerabilities and super-powers.

- Self-compassion has two aspects: the loving kindness and fierce loyal loving.

- Self-compassion allows us to accept that suffering is a part of the human condition.

- Self-compassion is associated with better emotional health, productivity and happiness and less fear, negativity and anger.

- Self-compassion is a skill that can be acquired through practise.

chapter 25

TRUTH AND TRUST

"Sometimes not getting what you want is a wonderful stroke of luck."

– Dalai Lama

There is a little story I love from Rick Hanson's book *Buddha's Brain*. Rick is going for a walk in the forest one afternoon and he finds himself staring into the eyes of an owl. The curious and wise bird stays very still, and Rick gets a sense of its wisdom and presence. He says to the bird, "I wish you well, I hope that you find what you need" and walks on. A few hundred metres ahead, he comes face-to-face with a busy little squirrel. There is a moment where they look at each other before it dashes away. Rick shares the same wish for the squirrel. Then he stops for a moment. The little squirrel is likely to be dinner for the owl. Rick ponders this conflict. By wishing the owl well, he is wishing, in a way, that the squirrel becomes his dinner. But then he realises that this is just life. He has no control over the outcome, but he can still wish each being well.

In this same way, we can choose to wish ourselves well. This is a choice, a practise and an option. We can hope for ourselves, because we are all worthy of success, love and dreams. We can choose to trust.

Trust is a part of our nature. Our innate survival mechanism is driven by the heart's hormonal system. Oxytocin is the hormone of love, trust and bonding. It is a key player in breastfeeding and the maternal/child bond, but men can produce it very well as well. Having a loving conversation, sharing a meal and making love all increase its supply to the body. It helps us relax. It allows us to become more intimate and surrender to connection.

Trust is something we build up. It is subtle and intuitive. It requires consistency, reliability, and truth — truth being a belief that is honest and accurate to reality. Trusting the truth in a world that is busy can be a challenge, especially when we are overwhelmed, stressed or in a state of anxiety and threat.

Truth lives in the body; the human body follows the principles of nature. Our personalities and beliefs can be held by society, but the body doesn't necessarily live by those rules. The rushing, the competition, the comparisons and the pressure are external factors that impact the body, but do not change its fundamental truths.

Your human life and the choices you make are unique to you. Your desires, your preferences and your beliefs are yours, you own them. They may have been shaped in part by where you were born, your family, your socioeconomic status or your education level, but you love what you love, you value what you value and you believe what you believe. It is as simple as that. The challenge is when we feel pressured to be a certain way, when we feel that we don't belong, when we are behaving in a way that doesn't feel right for us, or when we don't even feel like we know who we are, what we like and what we value.

Coming into the body and starting a reflective relationship with it is the start of unravelling the truth that lives within you. Over time and with practise you will then learn to trust this as a source of guidance and companionship. Trust is something I have relied upon, especially during tough times. It has seemed almost like an appeal for hope. When I was really struggling, I could turn trust into a mantra of sorts, and create a scaffold for myself in dark times. You can do this too.

To trust, we need to befriend. We need to de-armour ourselves. We need to be open to new possibilities. One of my favourite sayings that I used to share with patients is "there is no change without change". We do tend to do the same thing over and over, expecting a different result.

We must learn how to trust. Trust is a process, and so is change. Because we are dealing mainly with the nervous system (of the body, brain and heart) it takes time — more time than we would ideally like in a world that works off immediate gratification. This means we must celebrate and embrace the small wins and the small gains as we retrain our bodies to be well. If you can do this, you will see progress faster and the transformation will not be lost.

Learning to trust is vital to this work, but trust can never be hurried. Even though betrayal is a normal part of the human journey, some of us have been more betrayed than others. Take trust slowly if you need. You are always in charge of how you feel and what you trust. Stay open to what it feels like to lean into it. Trust in your own body is where you need to start.

WHEN YOU HAVE LOST TRUST IN YOURSELF

Over the past decade or so, I have witnessed an incredible rise in the number of people who have lost trust in their bodies. It is especially in those who have received a diagnosis of autoimmunity or cancer, but it can occur in other illnesses or mental health challenges as well. The rise of the 'internet expert' and the explosion of a knowledge-based culture has amplified the aloneness and confusion that can be felt with diagnoses such as these.

Cancer is often a silent disease. It doesn't often present with pain, especially in the early stages. Some people simply go to the doctor with another issue, then testing reveals an extraordinary and mind-blowingly unexpected diagnosis of cancer.

Autoimmunity on the other hand can be a protracted diagnostic situation. Often a person is feeling fatigued, inflamed and in pain. The elusive nature of autoimmunity is such that the underlying cause is that the immune system turns in on itself and starts attacking itself. The patient literally feels like they are under attack, and feels they are to blame or feels ashamed of it. The process to turn this around is beyond the scope of the book, but letting these illnesses become teachers, and learning to trust the body and its ability to heal (in addition to the treatment prescribed) is a potential avenue for care that often is left unexplored.

Exercise: Wishing Yourself Well Meditation

This is a very ancient meditation where we practise the skills of self-care, compassion for others — not only those we love — and to beings in general. If done daily for six weeks, this practise will transform your relationship with yourself and with life.

To begin, close your eyes. Sit comfortably with your feet flat on the floor and your spine straight. Relax your whole body. After you have read through the script, keep your eyes closed throughout the whole visualisation and bring your awareness inward. Without straining or concentrating, just relax and gently follow the instructions.

Take a deep breath in. And breathe out.

Receiving Loving-Kindness

Think of a person close to you who loves you very much. It could be someone from the past or the present, someone still in life or who has passed. Imagine that person standing on your right side, sending you their love. That person is sending you wishes for your health and safety, for your wellbeing and happiness. Feel the warm wishes and love coming from that person towards you.

Now bring to mind the same person or another person who cherishes you deeply. Imagine that person standing on your left side, sending you wishes for your wellness, for your health and safety, wellbeing and happiness. Feel the kindness and warmth coming to you from that person.

Now imagine that you are surrounded on all sides by all the people who love you and have loved you. Picture all your friends and loved ones surrounding you. They are sending you wishes for your health, safety, wellbeing and happiness. Bask in the warm wishes and love coming from all sides. You are filled and overflowing with warmth and love.

Sending Loving-Kindness to loved ones

Now bring your awareness back to the person standing on your right side. Begin to send the love that you feel back to that person. You and this person are similar. Just like you, they wish to be happy. Send all your love and warm wishes to that person.

Repeat the following phrase three times, silently: *May you live with ease, may you be happy, may you be free from pain.*

Now focus your awareness on the person standing on your left side. Begin to direct the love within you to that person. Send all your love and warmth to them. That person and you are alike. Just like you, that person wishes to have a good life.

Repeat the following phrase three times, silently: *Just as I wish to, may you be safe, may you be healthy, may you live with ease and happiness.*

Now picture another person you love, perhaps a relative or a friend. This person, like you, wishes to have a happy life. Send warm wishes to that person.

Repeat the following phrase three times, silently: *May your life be filled with happiness, health and wellbeing.*

Sending Loving-Kindness to neutral people

Now think of an acquaintance, someone you don't know very well and toward whom you do not have any particular feeling. You and this person are alike in your wish to have a good life.

Send all your wishes for wellbeing to that person, repeating the following phrase three times, silently: *Just as I wish to, may you also live with ease and happiness.*

Now recall another acquaintance toward whom you feel neutral. It could be a neighbour, a colleague or someone else that you see around but do not know very well. Like you, this person wishes to experience joy and wellbeing in their life.

Send all your good wishes to that person, repeating the following phrase three times, silently: *May you be happy, may you be healthy, may you be free from all pain.*

Sending Loving-Kindness to all living beings

Now expand your awareness and picture the whole globe in front of you as a little ball.

Send warm wishes to all living beings on the globe, who, like you, want to be happy.

Just as I wish to, may you live with ease, happiness, and good health.

Take a deep breath in. And breathe out. And another deep breath in and let it go.

Notice the state of your mind and how you feel after this meditation.

When you're ready, open your eyes.

chapter 26

PITFALLS AND SETBACKS

"People who have no vices have very few virtues."

– Abraham Lincoln

Flexibility and adaptability are the key to a long life. Flexibility in all arenas of life, body, heart and soul. Adaptation to internal and external changes is vital to our survival. But adaptation can be really hard, and it is likely that you will meet many challenges along the way. This chapter explores six common patterns that I commonly see in people who develop stress, anxiety or burnout. It is important to be mindful of these as you journey ahead, remembering that perfection is not the aim.

1. Hooked on busyness

"Beware the barrenness of a busy life."

– Socrates

When I was in fifth-year medical school, I was lucky enough to do a stint at the hospital in Port Vila, Vanuatu. We would start early, at 6:00am, and by midday we had done all the ward rounds, written up orders and admitted or discharged who we needed to. We had the afternoon free to rest, relax and study. We would return around 4:00pm to review the patients, check in with the nurses and finish what needed to be done.

In the gap, my friend and I would catch the ferry across to Iriki Island and lay on the beach, swim and read. Mangoes that fell off the tree around the corner would intermittently wash up in the tides. As the water lapped at our feet, we would simply reach down, peel another mango, and then wash our hands and face in the water again. Life was simple, sweet and quiet. We are biologically adapted to this kind of mellow afternoon, where we work for a little bit, then rest for a little bit.

Of course, this is nothing like what most of us do on a day-to-day basis. Modern life is hectic, and full of pressure. Stress and busyness have become an identity. We honour it, and we celebrate it in others as a sign of success. It is very common to become addicted to it ourselves as a sign of our ego and self-worth. At times we are rushing so much that we don't even know why we are rushing. Rushing has become so normal that it is even hard to stop rushing on the weekends.

It is important to realise that we can very easily become addicted to something without really noticing. We become trapped in a life of our own making. Mindless living can lead us in a direction that can be vastly different to how we had set out to live and somehow, we forget to check in and reflect. This latter point is common for those in burnout. Burnout does not have to be from over-work, it can be from doing the wrong kind of work, that doesn't suit our values, our dreams or our skills. It can be from a life that feels at odds with our deeper sense of who we are and how we would like to live.

Exercise: Hooked on a Feeling

If this sounds familiar, perhaps make a time to ponder this compulsion to busyness. What is it you are getting from rushing? Does it make you feel important? Does it make others think you are essential? Are other people's needs more important than your own? Is there some form of gain from staying in the pain? Do you feel bored otherwise? Have you normalised stress in your life so much that when you are not stressed you feel bored, unproductive, worthless or redundant?

2. Being Pollyanna

> *"Even a happy life cannot be without a measure of darkness, and the word happy would lose its meaning if it were not balanced by sadness. It is far better to take things as they come along with patience and equanimity."*
>
> – Carl Jung

Remember Pollyanna? That annoyingly cheesy, uber positive girl with rosy cheeks and a constant smile. The girl who could turn a violent storm into a rainbow.

We are always told to be positive, to look on the bright side, to find the silver lining, be grateful for what we have. Despite this being good advice at times, some people can use this unrealistic optimism as a block to their ability to look at their own suffering. Going straight to gratitude all the time can be a way of avoiding or ignoring the issues. By doing this as a habit, you can miss the vital information you need to build your own sense of self, and know who you are, what you value and what your boundaries are. This can lead to a perpetual cycle of stress and suffering, which can also be a kind of addiction — a representation of self-sabotage, fear of being seen, shame or low self-worth, or a sense that others deserve happiness, joy and relaxation but not you. This is a less obvious ego manifestation that often eludes our attention. It slips under the radar.

This kind of subtle ego is common in women but can be seen in men too. It tends to manifest in service-orientated people — workhorses, kind-hearted people, healers, empaths and Samaritans who always reflect on their good fortune, even when they feel overwhelmed by their workload. This ability to put a positive spin on things is often entrenched in their personality, but when it is at the expense of their own experience of life, their own ownership of happiness or their own mental and physical wellbeing, it becomes an unhelpful survival adaptation. It needs to be attended to so this person can have a more balanced approach to life and find their joy and shared humanity.

If we don't realise that ego is driving the whole process, it often repeats itself in a different job or a different relationship or a different circumstance. Because it isn't often discussed, people don't seek support for this.

Pollyannas tend to find getting angry very challenging. If we look at anger as a way of identifying boundaries, then Pollyannas tend to have a challenge asserting and maintaining their boundaries. This is often what is behind stress and burnout. Boundaries are an act of love. They bring clarity to a relationship, ownership of ourselves and an ability to get to know another person with dignity, respect and honour.

The inability to say no, to assert our boundaries and therefore to know and respect our own limits, is a hidden source of stress. It limits our control over how others may treat us, and therefore limits our own ability to care for ourselves and others. Pollyannas tend to over-care. They care for others at the expense of caring for themselves.

3. Avoiding the issues

"Choosing our own comfort over hard conversations
is the epitome of privilege, and it corrodes trust and moves us
away from meaningful and lasting change."

– Brené Brown.

Stress, anxiety and burnout can be both a cause and effect of a state of avoidance. This is where we avoid the hard conversations, and avoid looking in on ourselves to allow ourselves to become more real. Being avoidant means we trigger a coping style that is defined by denying what is really going on, dissociating ourselves from the issue and getting or keeping ourselves pre-occupied with something else. By always going into denial and pre-occupation, you can bypass the reality of the situation — say, the ongoing abuse of your time, your generosity or your inability to say no. Avoidants assume there is nothing that can be done to help the situation, so they don't ask for help or try to fix the issue. Avoidants have a knack of acting aloof, cool and competent, but they rarely identify the fear that sits below their patterned responses.

Becoming avoidant is not a personality trait. It is simply a self-protection mechanism that kicked in for whatever reason to help someone's internal nervous system cope with something that was distressing for them. This may lead to an inability to sit with discomfort. This in turn can lead to a pattern of being that is static and difficult to move through, as life and relationships fall into patterns that do not fully serve you.

The trick for the avoidants is to understand that these approaches to protection can stop them from fully coming into their aliveness; their protection mode is hindering their heart-led expressions. Avoidants need to start getting comfortable with the uncomfortable, rather than running away or pushing it away. This strategy is all about not wanting to feel, to pretend that they don't feel much or that whatever happened didn't impact them much.

Bypassing our challenges is very common and is hard to overcome, as we often feel rewarded for our ways of dealing with challenges. Others call us resilient, grateful, easy-going. Our ability to be non-reactive and cool under certain circumstances is revered. It is often difficult to talk to people who have developed such ways of behaving in life; they often feel resentful and confused as to why the framework that has worked for them for so long needs to be dismantled if they want to find a solution to their anxiety, stress and burnout. These are the people who feel bothered if you bring up their problems. They like to brush over themselves, and often feel like their issues are self-indulgent, frivolous or ridiculous.

Some people are masterful in disguise but are forever left wondering why they feel so fatigued, why their seemingly 'stress-related illness' like eczema, tension headaches or IBS doesn't go away, when they 'don't even feel stressed'. These people need to learn to sit with the pain of the relationships they are in, the relationship they have with themselves, and the illness they may have or the burden of work they may feel. The only way is for them is to take off their masks and truly embrace self-compassion, work on really engaging in the felt sense of the body and get themselves on the same page as they put others.

Avoidants are not comfortable with their fears. When they tune into their fears it can feel overwhelming. But fear is what drives us towards change and fear helps us navigate our way around life. Denying our stress, fear and vulnerability can be a driver for creating inbuilt limitations on our lives, leading to perpetuating the feelings of stress, anxiety and burnout that the person is so desperately trying to avoid. Avoidants tend to 'under-care' about what they want and how they can source joy and love and all the things that are antidotes to the stresses of life.

4. The stoic independent

"When there is no enemy within,
the enemies outside cannot hurt you."

– African proverb

Another common pattern that is seen in people who develop anxiety, stress and burnout is the stoic independent. This is someone who tends to hide their struggles, judges others for their overt emotional responses, never asks for help and can feel vulnerable when they are in need.

This hyper-independent adaptation to life is revered and rewarded in society. It is common in those who fear loss, or feel very vulnerable in connecting with their failures, insecurities and weaknesses. They defend against anyone seeing this, sometimes at all costs. This may mean isolating their hearts from others; not willing to be seen, just in case they are exposed. It may mean fighting to be everything for themselves so that they don't risk having to be dependent on anyone else.

Hyper-independence is a trauma response. We all have needs in life, from having food and shelter, to having a listening ear, a loving caregiver, a hug, a mentor, touch, silence, guidance and respect. Our caregivers, especially in these highly time pressured times, can fall short of our needs, and we may not be great at knowing what we need, asking for what we need or handling our needs when they are not met. So we all arrive in adulthood with unmet needs. These unmet needs often are a source of shame.

We often don't know how to meet these unmet needs on our own, so we end up wanting other people to meet them for us. But because we don't know how to ask for them to be met this can make for trouble. To start to become conscious that we do have these things, and that others do too, allows us to connect to each other and ourselves in a more humane and sensitive way. In a way, it is simply another aspect of our shared humanity.

Practically speaking, finding out how to assess and respond to our unmet needs is a part of learning how to re-parent ourselves in adult-hood. Re-parenting means that we can transform the relationship we have with ourselves and learn to be gentle and sincere, and to offer ourselves respect. Most people don't get the opportunity to do this, and they go around their worlds with an inability to ask for what they need. They retreat into themselves and rely only on themselves to be everything to everyone, except their deeper self.

5. Spiritual bypassing

> "The tendency to use spiritual ideas and practices to sidestep or avoid facing unresolved emotional issues, psychological wounds, and unfinished developmental tasks."

> – John Welwood

Spiritual bypassing is when a person uses spiritual practices and beliefs as a defense mechanism, rather than confronting or working through challenging issues, emotions and relationships. While it can sound like a way to protect your self, and bring calmness and peace in difficult times, it isn't very effective at resolving the issues and often leads to glossing over challenging issues. Fear of connection is at the root of survival adaptations. This makes sense, as they often come from our childhood or early adult experiences, where we may have felt that we had no other choice but to respond in such ways. Responding repeat-edly in this way makes the adaptations into patterns and for some, entrenched personality traits. To unravel from these and find new ways of connecting to yourself and the world, you need to learn to recognise them when they are at play and start the process of making room for a different way of responding to life.

Finding new ways to elicit safety in your social touch nervous system, and more ways to take charge of your autonomic nervous system and make room for the breath and the heart, can help to guide you into being more truthful inside yourself. Seeking silence, seeking a listening ear, even if it is just your own, can open you up to new possibilities and new ways of revealing who you truly are.

We all know our truth, it is unique to us. It is our resonance that we have with the planet, our world and our people. But we unconsciously hide behind these survival adaptations that mask our needs, our desires and our wisdom. Becoming anxious, or owning our fears, is one way of finding the gold that lives within.

Biologically we are driven for connection, but our wounds stop us from leaning into our lives. We retreat away from the very things that can help us feel both autonomous and accepted, or we become hooked on things — such as gratitude, chanting, yoga classes, meditation, marathon running or work — that allow us a quick fix to our discomfort, thereby bypassing the challenges that keep us on the same road of suffering we are forever trying to get off.

6. Shame

> "Shame is a soul-eating emotion."
>
> – Carl Jung

There are nine innate emotional states known to humans: fear, anger, shame, joy, disgust, surprise, acceptance, sadness and expectation. Anger, fear, joy and sadness are the most common and known aspects of human emotion, and our behaviour is driven by them. Shame is rarely spoken of.

Shame is thought to be intrinsic because it holds the ability to control the behaviour of another person or people quickly and effectively to make sure the group stays together. We all have it. Shame is our collective unspeakable.

We process most of our emotions when we are alone, but shame seems to need the power of community to dissipate. I have had the privilege of being in groups where someone has shared a story that has filled them with shame for years. The healing effect of having this witnessed, heard, received and seen by the group lifts their shame like a puff of smoke. It is amazing to watch. We all feel isolated when we feel our shame, but when we share it, our collective ability to simply hold it for others and wash it away is an elixir we didn't even know we had access to.

I know many people will find this daunting, but it is simply how the biology of shame works. If shame has a bigger role in your life than previously acknowledged, please consider group work. Groups have a profound way of shifting shame and can offer you the space to transform this tricky, sticky emotion more easily and quickly. If your natural inclination is to avoid groups at all costs, I implore you to re-consider. Shifting shame can be so hard on your own, but if you find the courage to connect and dare to share, it can help you let go of shame and find the aliveness and truth you crave.

Exercise: Being My Truth

Ask yourself:

- Are you being overly disciplined, even when that discipline is highly admired, such as health and wellness?

- Is there is a strictness at play, a rigidity?

- Can you be disciplined and playful too?

- Do you tend to go it alone, to not ask for support?

- Do you dismiss others' opinions as frivolous?

- When things get uncomfortable do you turn immediately to gratitude?

- When conversations get hard, do you like to change the line of discussion to something more cheerful?

- Are you the island (potentially a very successful island, but an isolated island all the same)?

- Does someone's support or kindness make you feel vulnerable and weak? Does it make you feel ashamed?

These are all signs that our survival patterns are at play. It is worth checking in with yourself for these attributes.

Our personality, skills or attributes can be the tickets to our success, but they can also make us rigid, hardened and fixated. Watch for these characteristics of your choices and relationships. It may be an avenue worth looking at so that you can find your freedom and joy.

chapter 27

THE WONDER WITHIN PLAYLIST

"Play is our brain's favorite way of learning"

– Diane Ackerman

A native American elder was once asked how she became so wise, so content and so respected. She answered: "In my heart there are two wolves, a wolf of love and a wolf of hate. The one who wins is the one I feed."

Play is a critical part of learning, a time where we surrender the rules, the conditioning and we give ourselves the freedom to make mistakes, to try new things and to challenge our old ways of doing things. In this next section, I ask you to dig deep, to use playfulness (despite any shyness or resistance) and to embrace your aliveness, for yourself. What you pay attention to grows. This is fundamental to how the brain grows, adapts and changes. This is so important for those with obsessional thinking or ruminating thinking. You are not your thoughts, but you do have the ability to change whether you feed them or not.

The wonder within is an adventure of a lifetime. But like all adventures, it will be brought home by planning, persistence and attention to detail. Knowing how to feed your thoughts, finding and savouring the good and discovering new ways of overcoming hurdles will help you expand your mindset and ultimately find your way toward the depths of your being. Anxiety, stress and burnout can be invitations to your unfurling and to accessing the wonder within. In the next section are 10 things you can add to your life's playlist to help you succeed and flourish as you dig deep and find your aliveness.

1. Practise is vital

> "Practise isn't the thing you do once you're good. It's the thing you do that makes you good."
>
> – Malcolm Gladwell

Leyton Hewitt, love him or hate him, was an Australian tennis champion. World number one at age 20, where he stayed for 80 weeks. He was renowned as having one of the best returns of serve in the history of the game. He was passionate, fiery and bold; you couldn't fault him for energy and commitment.

His tennis career was plagued with injury. After several hip surgeries, he needed to totally reform his play to manage future injury recurrence. Under the guidance of sports physiotherapy and exercise physiology, he had to retrain his brain and body.

When people become masters of a skill, be they a concert violinist, an elite sportsperson, a renowned yogi or a linguist who can speak five languages, the area in their brain's cortex become extremely refined, denser and plumper than those who are more pedestrian in their skills. I can imagine that Hewitt's motor cortex would have been a little swollen compared to mine. He had to retrain the automation that had become so expert and commonplace for him. This is not an easy thing to do. It requires great commitment, focus and most importantly, repetition.

It is thought to take 10,000 repetitions to fully retrain a trained brain. For those of us who are trained in fear-based thinking, highly skilled in looking at the negatives and profoundly accomplished in making the future look like a catastrophe, we will need to bring in trust 10,000 times. Remember to focus on our breath 10,000 times. Focus deeply into our hearts 10,000 times, and tell ourselves how much we love ourselves 10,000 times.

We tend to embrace training when we do something big, like set out to run a marathon. We know that if we've just sat on the couch for six months, then running 15 kilometres on the first training day is not achievable. But we don't seem to have the same respect for the way emotional neuronal connections work and re-establish themselves through brain, body and heart-based skills in other areas of refinement.

The 10,000 repetitions required is not to put you off. You will experience much improvement, joy and peace along the way. But it does serve to remind you to take it easy on yourself, keep your expectations in check and make sure you stay dedicated to your greatest adventure: befriending your stunning, gorgeous, mysterious, loving human heart.

Creating a logbook of practise can help you bring this into a daily opportunity for change. Remember, anything can be seen as practise:

- A long slow deep breath at a traffic light will set the cascade of relaxation chemicals through your body.

- Washing the dishes as you mindfully and slowly watch your breath.

- A yoga class.

- A five-minute meditation session.

- A walk in nature.

- Watching a sunrise or a sunset.

- Listening to your favourite piece of music.

I see a lot of people with anxiety or stress who, even though they have experienced some relief from some of the exercises they have been shown, continue to belittle them as a solution. The first part of the journey is by far the hardest. Everything in your neurons and brain is pulling back to the stress that you have normalised. But to resist change is to remain in pain. You are the boss of your body and you are the boss of your life, even if at times it doesn't feel that way.

You might need a lot of help to get you through the first stages of change. You might need a counsellor, a psychologist, a coach or a GP. You might need a yoga class, meditation course, apps such as Insight Timer, or to set reminders in your phone.

Set up a small space in your house to go to. Buy yourself a new set of runners and a rain jacket so you can walk in any weather. As part of your commitment to yourself and to maximise your ability to achieve, reach out for support.

As time goes on the skills will become part of your second nature, and you may not need to go to so many classes or appointments to maintain your gains.

2. Savour the good

"The trouble is, you think you have time."

– Buddha

Negativity bias is a part of our natural survival biology. It is in our survival favour to focus on what went wrong more than what went right. If we were staring at the beautiful sunset at the same time as we could see a wild bear approaching us, we would wind up dead!

We are all familiar with how this goes. Imagine you spend days writing a speech to present to your peers, you do a great performance and everybody comes up afterwards and sings your praises. You feel relieved, proud and really happy with how it went. But as you walk back to your table you overhear one person mocking the speech. You are instantly sent into a whirlwind of negativity. You suddenly feel like an idiot, you feel humiliated, and all you can now think of is replaying the words of the critic back inside your own mind.

It isn't only you who does this. The example above actually happened to me during a keynote speech. When I heard a peer mocking me, I was instantly shattered. From elation to devastation — one comment led me to disregarding all the opinions of all the other people in that crowded room. I drove home that evening, vowing I would never sign up to do that again.

This is how we are all wired. It has been shown that we need nine positive comments for every one negative. To remedy this, we need to consciously savour the positives, and even relish in them. This turns the amplitude up on the para-sympathetic nervous system. It is like fertiliser that helps it grow stronger.

Savouring the positive is something we can all do, but it isn't automatic. It needs to be deliberate and practiced. It is a choice. By doing this, we actively heal the wounds inflicted on us by our excessive negative feedback system. The more you can practise savouring the good, the easier and more tilted towards the positive you will become.

Highlighting the positive is a way to give yourself a reality check. We unconsciously lean towards everything that is wrong in the world, where in fact, a lot of things go right for us all the time.

We notice when things go wrong. When we wake up in the morning, go to turn on the heater and the power is out and the kettle won't work. When we get in our car, and a tree is over the road. When we are late for work and miss an important meeting. We start pulling our hair out — if only we could start this day all over, because nothing is going right! Little did we appreciate the day before, when we were warm, sitting there with our hot coffee and newspaper, the traffic to work was a breeze and we nailed the presentation and won the account!

Savouring the positives can mean more than just diverting our attention away from the negative and coming back into balance. It can also be something we can do for ourselves that helps to intensify the lovely aspects of our lives.

I am a chronic overachiever. Yep, I said it! For a long time I wasn't aware of it, because a lot of doctors are chronic overachievers. So I didn't really notice. I would never stop to tune into what I had achieved. I would get through a milestone, like opening a new clinic, and literally the next day start working towards another goal. It was like, tick … next!

It wasn't that I wasn't proud of what I had done, I just didn't think to truly reflect on all the things that had led to this moment. I didn't reflect on my good fortune, or on those who helped me along the way, or my hard work or my success. So many wonderful things occurred, and they were not given the dues they deserved.

I was so hopeless at savouring that I would feel stressed when I was on holidays, just in case I wasn't enjoying myself enough. I put too much pressure on the actual fun meter and forgot to have fun. Savouring has taught me to slow down, to reflect, to bring in my gratitude, my blessings. It has also allowed me to connect with how much support I receive. Savouring helps us be humble, gracious and mindful.

Let's start focusing on the positives.

Exercise: Time to Savour

Take a moment to sit quietly in a comfortable place. Reflect on a time you felt really good about something you did or achieved. It could be that you cooked a meal for someone in need, gave up a vice that wasn't healthy for you, volunteered at the local school for a morning, got praise for an assignment you handed in, or said yes to something that challenged you.

Take some time to feel the moment in time as if it is happening right now. Look around and reflect on how you feel, the praise, the gratefulness or the esteem that comes from doing something esteemed. See if you can amplify the feeling. Make a concerted effort to grow this feeling. Consider your good fortune, or luck, the support of those around you, your determination, your efforts or your thoughtfulness.

If those pesky thoughts of 'not good enough' are coming in during this reflection, see if you can watch them, and still go on and offer yourself some savouring. Linger longer with the nice states of mind and heart that you are feeling. Amplify, savour, embellish. Why not?

3. Internalise the positive

> "If you don't like the road you're walking, start paving
> another one."
>
> – Dolly Parton

You can turn positive thoughts into positive experiences. Thoughts are brain energy, and experiences bring them into the body.

When someone says something nice about you, don't rush over it. Take it in. Make their nice reflection into an experience. Savour it, bring it into your heart space and hold it. Let it infuse into your heart and allow that feeling to spread throughout your body from there.

When you do something kind or you help someone in some way, instead of passing over this experience as a given, take it in. Give yourself credit and make it a tactile experience.

When you finish a task, savour the moment and take it inside you. You have achieved something, you have worked hard, persisted, and gotten over procrastination. Savour the experience of finishing.

You can do this for little things too: a cute child, a beautiful flower, a hug, a stunning bite of dessert. Open to the positives and really embellish them. Stay with these moments for 10 to 30 seconds at least. In the moments that are more monumental, such as finishing a big project, make sure you celebrate, rest, relax and reward yourself. Take in the accomplishment, take in the platitudes.

By doing this you are recreating positive pathways in your neurons and strengthening the memories that will help you balance the positives and the negatives. Remember, neurons that fire together wire together. The stronger we make the positives, the less burdensome the negatives will become. By doing this, we lower our stress hormone cortisol and increase oxytocin. We lower adrenaline and increase dopamine. We have the power to do this — if not now, when?

4. Play with pronoia

"Shine like the whole universe is yours."

– Rumi

When I was first anxious, I felt very paranoid. I was overly concerned about what other people thought of me and I was paranoid about bad things happening to me. Paranoia is the illogical feeling that people are out to get you. It is essentially a state of extreme mistrust of the world and of others. This is not a natural state, nor is it healthy. We can think ourselves into paranoia, like how conspiracy theories work as a collective groupthink.

Pronoia is essentially the opposite of paranoia. Pronoia is where we start to believe that the universe and all the people in our lives are here to support us, that they all wish us well, think well of us and are all colluding to help us be happy.

Playing with the concept of pronoia can be very illuminating, especially if you are in a trap of always thinking people think poorly of you, or that bad things are more likely to happen. I encourage you to give it a go.

Exercise: The World Is On Your Side

Try on the concept of pronoia for a day. Imagine that everyone you meet has your best interests at heart. Even if you come into a form of conflict or disagreement, stay with pronoia as the lens you see this through. Wherever you go, take pronoia with you.

- What do you notice?

- How is the world different?

- Did you feel better or worse?

- Do you feel more optimistic or not?

- Do you feel more confident?

- Did it help you think differently of other people?

5. The power of nature

"Into the forest I go to lose my mind and find my soul."

– John Muir

The natural world is more than a place of beauty. Our environment alters the chemicals released inside our brains and bodies. When we are surrounded by trees, they have a resonance, which attunes with our resonance. We connect to them and they connect to us. We breathe out CO_2 and they breathe it in. They make oxygen, and we breathe it in.

Like humans, trees communicate with each other, using their extensive and deep root systems. Suzanne Simard, a Canadian forest ecologist, discovered that older trees share resources with younger trees (as opposed to the dominant view that larger trees have a competitive advantage over saplings) and furthermore, that trees communicate with the same neuro-transmitters found in the human brain. Professor Simard found that the processes that support a well-functioning forest mirror the maps of the human brain. She named the mature hub trees 'Mother Trees'. These trees parent and share their wisdom in a mutual and reciprocal way. This also mirrors what we acknowledge to be true of fully flourishing human ecosystems.

If we consider the Industrial Revolution as the first major urbanisation, humans as a species resided in natural environments for nearly 99.99 per cent of the past five million years. Our biology, physiology and neurology has evolved and adapted to nature, which is why nature is so healing for us and helps the body re-establish a calmness inside itself. Now we are living through the most rapid changes in technology in human history. Australians are working amongst the longest hours in the world, and excessive screen time is adding to the burden of nature deprivation seen amongst our community.

Shinrin-yoku, also known as forest bathing, involves utilising the positive effects of trees and nature to re-establish a balance in the human physiology — literally using the trees as medicine. It has been associated with multiple health benefits, such as an improvement in the rate of healing post operatively and increased immunity, including a rise in natural killer cells, which help protect the body against cancer.

People have less anxiety and depression after being exposed to nature. One study found that 120 minutes per week is all that is needed to elicit this response; the time can be taken in 20-minute increments or all at once.

Nature, especially where there are bodies of water, also exposes us to a greater amount of negative ions. Negative ions are charged atoms that have an increased energy. This increase of chemical energy has a positive effect on your mental health. Waterfalls, oceans and babbling streams all emit higher levels of negative ions, whereas the air found in most office buildings has little to no negative ions.

Most of us inherently know that we feel better after a walk, or when we take a weekend out of the city. When you are more intentional about your time in nature you can amplify its effects.

Exercise: Nature Fix

Try walking slowly through the bush, a garden or any green space. Breathe in the smells and listen for the noises, near and far. Even listen to the silence and bring in the vibrations inside your body. Tune in and see if your vibrational energy changes in the forest. Try hugging a tree or telling a tree all your problems. Lie on the grass and tune into the feeling of having the earth beneath you. See if you can feel her support, perhaps you might even feel her pulse.

Imagine the ground beneath you connected via the roots of all the surrounding trees. Most of the trees you will walk amongst are older that you, and depending on where you are, they might be older than your great-grandparents. Imagine what they have seen.

After your walk, reflect on how you feel. Use your imagination, your wonder and your awe to guide you into new ways of thinking, trusting, connecting and embracing the world that you are a part of. If you are stressed, anxious or burnt out, do yourself a favour and get up close and personal with a forest.

6. Fake it until you make it

"Believe you can and you are halfway there."

– Theodore Roosevelt.

The reality of this is quite unbelievable. In many ways the reality we create for ourselves is unique to us — we have more power over our lives than we give ourselves credit for. Faking it until you make it is all about resetting your nervous system and using your imagination to bring you into a new reality.

When you are in a state of stress, anxiety or burnout it is difficult to feel new emotions. I remember the feeling of flatness and the inability to find joy. Faking it until you make it is a way of seeking and finding joy.

Think back to the stick versus the snake story in Part 2. If we see a stick on the ground and think it is a snake, our fear response has the same intensity as if we actually saw a snake on the ground. Faking it is our way of reversing this and tricking our brain and nervous system to suit our healing.

Laughter yoga and laughter therapy are excellent resources you might turn to. You could also watch a funny movie, even if you only laugh once. Even putting your arms up in the air in the victory signal has a positive effect on the mind.

Researchers in the 1970s showed that changing your body posture changes your mindset. Try it now. Stand up, take three big deep breaths in and out through your nose. Put your hands high up in the air, like you are in a victory pose. Imagine yourself winning a race or standing on top of a mountain. Now try to feel angry. Now try to feel depressed. Go on, try harder.

Now try to feel joy. Feel it deep within. Imagine feeling joy pumping through your heart and body. Keep your arms up in the air. Feel it, breathe it in. You are now pure joy and nothing else. Imagine yourself laughing, just because you are alive.

Bring joy in, nobody cares if you fake it! Fake joy… and watch and wait to see what happens.

Just as putting your hands up in the air automatically brings a sense of aliveness to the body, slumping over and shrugging your shoulders makes it harder to feel joy. The slumping body position is associated with depression. Try it yourself. See what a difference your body posture makes to your instantaneous emotions.

7. Share your story

> "There is no greater agony than bearing an untold story
> inside you."
>
> – Maya Angelou

When we suffer, we contract. It is a natural response to hardship and struggle. We make ourselves small and less significant, which gives us a false sense of safety. When we share our pains and sufferings with others we open up, we expand into the other person's space. And because we are all wired for storytelling and we are all mirrors for each other, this act of sharing our story is profoundly healing for not only ourselves but for the listener too. I can't tell you how many times I would sit and listen to a person tell their story, only to witness in amazement the similarities we shared as we journeyed through our lives. How they struggled with the same things I struggled with. It was so humbling, inspiring and comforting to witness this, to support another person just by listening and reflecting and offering space and time to heal. I am so lucky to play this role in people's lives as it is so healing for me too.

By finding the courage to share your story, you never realise how powerful it can be to the person listening and the potential ramifications that this may have on your life and the lives of people you don't even know.

Shame lives in silence. The more we hold onto our silence, the more shame grows and festers. Be brave and share.

8. Ask for help

"Life shrinks or expands according to one's courage."

–Anais Nin

Asking for help is akin to sharing, as asking for help allows you to soften into yourself, but also offers the person being asked to open their heart too. Asking for support is courageous and it offers a heart-opening experience for both people. Our healing is a collective experience, one that offers hope not only to ourselves but to others too.

It can be hard for some people to seek help when times are tough, especially for the avoidants, the Pollyannas and the hyper-independents. Somewhere, somehow along the way, asking for help was not seen as the right thing to do, whether it simply wasn't there, it felt like they were being bothersome, or whether it felt like the caring was actually making things worse.

The way we are wired means that social support is a vital ingredient to personal growth. Whether via a mentor, a friend, a work colleague or a paid counsellor, sharing our story and seeking help can have an inordinate influence on our ability to reveal ourselves, learn about our deeper connections and gather more skills needed along the ride we all call life.

When we are anxious, stressed or burnt out we often lose perspective on our issues. We are at risk of apathy, have low motivation and quite simply can't muster any new ideas to support ourselves. As we let others in, we can use their perspective to help build up our own capacity again.

Be bold and get supported.

9. Altruism

> "The more you nurture a feeling of kindness,
> the happier and calmer you will be."
>
> – Dalai Lama

Small acts of kindness, generosity and giving are associated with better mental health. It seems we are hardwired for altruism. Themes of competitiveness and survival of the fittest run through our culture, but this behaviour is cultural conditioning, not a biological imperative. Generosity is thought to be associated with greater social success and therefore survival — and its real benefit is more to the giver than the receiver.

In fact, generosity may increase your life span. The John Templeton Foundation commissioned the University of California, Berkeley to write a white paper on the topic of The Science of Generosity. This paper shows that multiple studies have demonstrated the positive consequences of generosity, which may include an improvement in a person's mental and physical health, and found generosity was a contributing factor in potentially increasing a person's longevity. Another study[16] which followed 2,700 people over 10 years found that men who regularly did volunteer work had death rates 2.5 times lower than those who didn't. Generosity reduces stress and enriches a person's sense of purpose.

In times of anxiety, stress and burnout, a great way to get out of ourselves is to think about what we can do for others. Sometimes people think too big when it comes to kindness. Little acts can have a big impact — things like writing a little note of love and putting it in a lunchbox, making someone else's bed, making someone dinner or even letting people into traffic.

Being generous is a state of mind that helps us bring people closer to us, and in turn we reap the benefits. If you are already adept at these small acts of kindness, you may instead focus on turning the acts of kindness inwards or learning how to accept acts of kindness from others.

It may be as simple as recognising how much kindness and generosity you already offer the world. Be realistic about what you can do. Start small, look outward and put kindness and generosity into your recipe for health and longevity.

10. Seek awe

> "[They] who can no longer pause to wonder and stand rapt in awe, is as good as dead: [their] eyes are closed."

> – Albert Einstein

In many ways awe can be seen as an altered state. Awe shifts our attention away from ourselves and onto something that is beyond our usual experience. It can make us feel like we are a part of something greater, and it is associated with generosity, open-mindedness and wonder.

Awe is a complex emotion and unlike other emotions can be either positive or negative. Psychologists Dacher Keltner and Johnathon

Haidt consider awe to have two aspects: a feeling of vastness, in combination with a need for accommodation. Awe feels big as well as intimate. The experience of it challenges our sense of normality and exceeds our expectations so much that there is a need to realign ourselves with a new normal. The two psychologists went on to confer that awe is associated with a feeling of smallness of self and a feeling of greater connectedness.

When we are stressed, anxious or in burnout, the experience of awe can help us to dramatically shift our focus in a new direction. Awe can be so impressive that it can be the impetus to make changes and to turn the corner towards health, wellness and a greater sense of connectedness to your life, the world and to others.

Perspective is often difficult to find in times of stress and anxiety. By finding awe we can set ourselves up for a transformation of our own neurology so that we can start to shift the tide in the opposite direction. Awe can be so powerful it can literally change your life.

Seeking awe is not a common prescription from a GP, but I hope one day it will be. The combination of excessive workload, anxiety, disconnection and nature deprivation means awe is in short supply.

As a reformed stress-head and anxiety sufferer, awe has changed me. Sitting on a mountain top, or on a rock that has been there for 350 million years, or walking the perimeter of Uluru, or looking up at the night sky in the middle of the desert, all gave me the opportunity to be completely metamorphosised.

If you are at the bottom of the barrel, staring out at the world with pain and suffering in your heart, awe can offer you the most dramatic opening for transcendence. Seek awe. Run towards it. It is there for the taking.

START WITH ONE MINUTE

These tools are all within our grasp, any time we choose to use them. Often when we feel anxious and stressed, we don't feel like turning to them. We don't feel like sitting on top of a mountain, we don't feel like putting our arms in the air, we don't feel like savouring the positives or faking joy or being altruistic. When your body and nervous system is so rundown that it expresses stress and anxiety as a normal response to life, you are not going to feel like doing these things.

But that doesn't mean you shouldn't do them. Often, we don't feel like going for a walk, but when we do go for a walk, we feel better. The same is true here. So, in the famous words of a Nike ad campaign… just do it.

Start with a minute. Everyone has that.

Make a commitment to practise one thing from this book for one minute a day for one week.

Set a timer for one minute and put an alert in your phone. If this is already something you do, double the time commitment, or do it a couple of times per day. Trusting the friendship between yourself and your emotions is vital in committing to a new way of living life.

EPILOGUE

The power of the whole is beyond a concept. It is essentially the foundation of all that we know. Everything in science comes back to the whole, everything in spirituality, everything in psychology, sociology and physiology. We are limited only by our obsession with pulling things apart and failing to put them back together.

We are more than the sum of our parts. We are integrally one with the universe. This isn't mysticism, this is reality. The more we play with and work towards accepting truth, mystery and everything in between, the better we can cope with the challenges of living this human life.

Stress, anxiety and burnout are the body's way of asking for change. They are the body's way of speaking; the emotional and physical response felt at the edge of its adaptation. Their expression has been simmering for a lot longer than you have realised.

We are all incredibly resilient. Many of us put up with challenges for longer than we ideally should for a whole raft of different reasons. We balance family, work, life, illness and relationships. But despite this incredible resilience we have, we all have the incredible power to make change too. Making changes can be hard, because 'our world' doesn't always seem to support it, but we have everything we need inside us to do it anyway.

This book is a playbook, filled with concepts that can and will blow your mind, and take you to a new level of understanding the most important thing there is to understand: yourself. How you work, how you relate, how you belong, how you love. Challenges and changes are rarely comfortable, but they are definitely doable.

You are never alone in this. You share your humanity with billions of others and you have so many untapped resources that live within. With a bit of practise and a loving commitment to your lived life, these skills can become stronger, more accessible and more enjoyable.

I hope you have gained some access to the wonder that lives within you.

I hope that you can find more pathways to your delicate, fierce and courageous heart.

I truly want to wish my fellow travellers well.

In the words of Gabor Mate, a Canadian physician and author, who writes extensively on healing trauma, "the fundamental healing agent is the alchemical transformation of our internal identity". When we transform, when we take on the change, we change our physiology to heal.

In a Lakota tribe in the US, when someone gets ill, it is not seen as an individual event but a collective one. They see illness as a representation of a social fracture in their culture and will search for the underlying causes or imbalances that may be at play. The community will gather with the person who is ill and be thankful that they have provided an opportunity to look within their society for issues that may need addressing. This interpretation of illness is vastly different from our society's understanding.

Can we be brave enough to take another look at the reality we are all living in?

Can we find the courage to broaden our perspective and learn from our pain?

Can we claim this opportunity to find a new way of healing?

I think we can.

The Wonder Within is my invitation to you to find your aliveness, to live your life with vitality, connection and a massive dose of whole-heartedness.

Be well, find awe and never forget: breathe your pants off!

NOTES

1   Peabody, F W. The care of the patient. *Journal of the American Medical Association*. 1927.

2   Egolf, B, Lasker, J, Wolf, S, and Potvin, L. The Roseto effect: a 50-year comparison of mortality rates. *Am J Public Health*. August 1992.

3   Valtorta, N K, et al. Loneliness and social isolation as risk factors for coronary heart disease and stroke: systematic review and meta-analysis of longitudinal observational studies. *Heart*. 2016 Volume 102 issue 13.

4   Almeida, D. M., Charles, S. T., Mogle, J., Drewelies, J., Aldwin, C. M., Spiro, A. III, & Gerstorf, D. Charting adult development through (historically changing) daily stress processes. *American Psychologist*. May-June 2020.

5   Sinnya S, De'Ambrosis B. Stress and melanoma: increasing the evidence towards a causal basis. *Arch Dermatol Res*. November 2013.

6   S K.H. Aung, H. Fay and R.F.Hobbs. Traditional Chinese Medicine as a Basis for Treating Psychiatric Disorders: A Review of Theory with Illustrative Cases. *Med Acupunct*. December 2013.

7   Planès S, Villier C and Mallaret M.. The nocebo effect of drugs. *Pharmacology Research & Perspectives*. 2016.

8   Two-way communication between the heart and the brain: Significance of time within the cardiac cycle March 1978 American Psychologist 33(2):99-113

9   Wölk, C., Velden, M., Zimmermann, U., & Krug, S. The interrelation between phasic blood pressure and heart rate changes in the context of the "baroreceptor hypothesis." *Journal of Psychophysiology. 1989*.

10 Davidson, R J, and Lutz, A. Buddha's Brain: Neuroplasticity and Meditation. *IEEE Signal Process Magazine*. January 2008.

11 Kolk, B. PTSD and the nature of trauma. *Dialogues in clinical neuroscience*. March 2010

12 AA Lima et al. The impact of tonic immobility reaction on the prognosis of PTSD. *Journal of psychiatric research* Volume 44 no 4. 2010.

13 Davidson, R J, and McEwen, B S. Social influences on neuroplasticity: Stress and interventions to promote well-being. *Nature Neuroscience*. April 2012.

14 Valk S et al. Structural plasticity of the social brain: differential change after socio-affective and cognitive mental training. *Science Advances*. Vol 3, issue 10. October 2017.

15 The Trap podcast hosted by Jess Hill. Episode 8. *Government, Policy and Power.*

16 Luoh, M and Regula Herzog, A. Individual Consequences of Volunteer and Paid Work in Old Age: Health and Mortality. *Journal of Health and Social Behavior*, vol. 43, no. 4, 2002.

CONNECT WITH ME

If you have found a connection within these words, and feel like sharing, I would love to hear from you about what resonated for you. Did anything challenge you, change you or inspire you?

If you are keen to know more, experience more and explore your inner world a little more, there are many ways we can continue to inspire each other and work together.

Make sure you head to www.theholisticgp.com.au to experience some of the exercises and meditations as audio immersions. You can listen to them as often as you like. There is also an opportunity to join the community to receive information about upcoming events, programs and immersions.

Instagram:@theholisticgp

Facebook: theholisticgp

LinkedIn: Dr Michelle Woolhouse

FURTHER READING

As well as scientific papers and formal reference books, there have been innumerable books, lectures, TED talks, podcasts and more that have informed my practice and this book. I have included this list for you to explore if you want to read more on this topic.

All the Rage: Buddhist wisdom on anger and acceptance. Contributors include Thich Nhat Hanh, Sharon Salzberg, Jack Kornfield, Noah Levine, Sylvia Boorstein and many more.

Anam Cara: Spiritual wisdom from the Celtic World by John O'Donohue

Atomic Habits: An easy and proven way to build good habits and break bad ones by James Clear

Brain Rules: 12 principles for surviving and thriving at work, home and school by John Medina

Buddha's Brain: The practical neuroscience of happiness, love and wisdom by Rick Hanson and Richard Mendius

Comfortable with Uncertainty: 108 teachings on cultivating fearlessness and compassion by Pema Chondron

Dare to Lead by Brene Brown

Full Catastrophe Living: How to cope with stress, pain and illness using mindfulness meditation by Jon Kabat Zinn

Getting Past Your Past: Take control of your life with self-help techniques from EMDR therapy by Francine Shapiro

Heart: A history by Sandeep Jauhar

Heart-Math Solution by Doc Childre and Howard Martin

Love, Medicine and Miracles by Bernie Seigel

261

Mindset: Change the way you think to fulfil your potential by Dr Carol Dweck

Mindsight: Change your brain and your life by Daniel Seigel

Molecules of Emotion: The science behind mind-body medicine by Candice Pert

On-Being podcast with Krista Tippett: A podcast on immersive conversations and explorations into the art of living.

Oneness With All Life: Awaken to a life of purpose and presence by Eckhart Tolle

Self-compassion: Stop beating yourself up and leave insecurity behind by Dr Kristin Neff

Softwired: How the new science of brain plasticity can change your life by Michael Merzenich

The Inner Self: The joy of discovering who we really are by Hugh Mackay

The Force of Kindness: Change your life with love and compassion by Sharon Salzberg

The Pocket Guide to the Polyvagal Theory: The transformative power of feeling safe by Stephen Porges

The Female Brain by Louann Brizendine MD

The Courage to be Disliked by Ichiro Kishimi and Fumitake Koga

The Essence of Health: the seven pillars of wellbeing by Dr Craig Hassed

The Brain's Way of Healing: Remarkable discoveries and recoveries from the frontiers of neuroplasticity by Norman Doidge

The Body Keeps the Score: Mind, brain and body in the transformation of trauma by Bessel Van Der Kolk

The Science of Happiness: How our brains make us happy and what we can do to get happier by Stefan Klein

The Brain that Changes Itself: Stories of personal triumph from the frontiers of brain science by Norma Doidge

The Five Things We Cannot Change: and the happiness we find by embracing them by David Richo

The Tao of Physics: An exploration of the parallels between modern physics and eastern mysticism by Fritjof Capra.

Touch: The science of the sense that makes us human by David J. Linden

When The Body Says No: The hidden cost of stress by Dr Gabor Mate

ABOUT THE AUTHOR

Dr Michelle Woolhouse is a holistic doctor and integrative health GP. She is also a podcaster, lecturer, keynote speaker and workshop facilitator.

Her philosophy is that health care should focus on the person as a whole, and address the physical, psychological, social and spiritual wellbeing of the individual.

A GP for more than 20 years, Dr Woolhouse also has post-graduate training in hypnotherapy, nutritional medicine, acupuncture and mind-body medicine. She draws on conventional Western medicine, complementary medicine and therapies, modern science and the wisdom of the ancients in her approach. She has an in-depth understanding of the underlying cause of diseases and in the healing principles of the body from an energetic, biochemical and structural level.

Dr Woolhouse is a fellow of the Royal Australian College of General Practitioners, the Australasian College of Nutritional and Environmental Medicine (ACNEM) and the Australasian Society of Lifestyle Medicine. She is a frequent lecturer and mentor for GP registrars and doctors and the founding medical director of Vive.ly, an innovative online tech platform aiming to transform the delivery of chronic disease management.

She is a host of the Blackmores Institute podcast Fx-Medicine. She previously co-founded and co-hosted award-winning health podcast The Good Doctors and is a faculty member and ambassador for ACNEM. She is also a keynote speaker in the arena of holistic health and anxiety and stress management, and the facilitator of health and empowerment immersions for women (www.theholisticgp.com.au). She won the National Institute of Integrative Medicine Lifetime commitment award for services to integrative medicine.

She has spent the last few years winding back the build-up of stress in her life after burning out from founding and running the innovative integrative general practice.

Dr Woolhouse has always had to battle her own anxiety and stresses, being a high achiever with a formidable inner critic. She has invested in freeing herself from the prison of her own making and seeks to find her own individual sense of aliveness through nature, presence, deep connection, growth and testing the boundaries. She was born an optimist and is forever seeking new ways to express the lifeforce that flows within her. Never content with saying no and sitting on the sidelines watching on, she is a fully engaged member of the human race, trying to be the best version of herself that she can be and seeking to find connection with the energetic force than we all share, we all belong to and we all seek to intimately know.

Dr Woolhouse is well and truly back from the depths of despair and transforming her lived experience, with freshness, newness and a big yes when required! She believes we are all on a kind of Hero's Journey, all reaching different peaks at different times, where joys and the sorrows equally light the way. She is committed to sharing her wisdom, her life lessons and her whole person medicine, so that people can feel the shared humanity that supported her so tenderly along the way.

Dr Woolhouse runs wellness immersions and online support groups. She is passionate about bringing holistic, integrative and lifestyle medicine into the laps of all the beautiful humans she shares the planet with.

Publications, Media and Ambassadorship

https://www.researchgate.net/profile/Michelle-Woolhouse

https://www.fxmedicine.com.au/users/michellewoolhouse

https://www.acnem.org/faculty/dr-michelle-woolhouse/

https://www.vively.com.au/team

Lightning Source UK Ltd.
Milton Keynes UK
UKHW010947281122
412977UK00004B/347